A Handbook of

NATURAL REMEDIES FOR COMMON AILMENTS

Books by Linda Clark:

Stay Young Longer
Get Well Naturally
Secrets of Health and Beauty
Are you Radioactive? How to Protect Yourself.
Color Therapy
Handbook of Natural Remedies for Common Ailments
Rejuvenation
Know Your Nutrition
Be Slim *and* Healthy
Health, Youth and Beauty Through Color Breathing (With Yvonne Martine)
Help Yourself to Health (a metaphysical book)
Face Improvement Through Exercise and Nutrition
The Best of Linda Clark (an Anthology)
Beauty Q&A. (With Kay Lee)

To find any of these books, please inquire at your health store, book store, or library.

A Handbook of
NATURAL REMEDIES FOR COMMON AILMENTS

by Linda Clark, M.A.

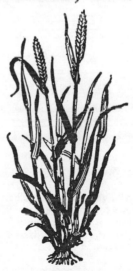

The Devin-Adair Company
Old Greenwich, Connecticut

Library of Congress Catalog Card Number: 75-13349
ISBN: 0-8159-5710-6

Printed in the United States of America

CONTENTS

A Note to the Reader

Many people are suffering from various ailments these days and need all the help they can find. Although these people share some of the same disturbances, they do not, of course, share them all. The following ailments are discussed for the benefit of those who *do* suffer from them. Those who do not, can pass them by, thank their lucky stars they are not so afflicted, and proceed to the discussion of disturbances which do plague them. Because diabetes is a doctor-controlled disease, it will not be covered in this book. If you have it, work with your doctor.

1: ARE YOU WELL?

This is a book dedicated to helping you get well. A completely well person is an exception today. Almost everyone has *something* wrong, either an outright disease or one or more small complaints such as headaches, fatigue, vague aches or pains. One young girl, just ready for college, told me, "I feel only half alive." This feeling is surprisingly common. Everyone would apparently like to have more vigor as well as get rid of ailments, large or small. So this book will deal with the most common illnesses experienced by the majority of people, telling how they may be handled naturally and, let's hope, providing some help for you, the reader.

As a reporter I wish to make it clear that I will not prescribe or even recommend the various natural treatments I will mention for each ailment. I will, however, *report* the remedies I have found which have helped others, quoting the sources where I have found the information. I do not intend to limit these remedies to any one field. Nature works through all systems of healing and we should use the good from all sources, how-

1

ever unorthodox, including nutrition, herbs, color therapy, homeopathy, osteopathy, chiropractic, or such things as reflexology and do-it-yourself acupuncture—known as contact therapy or acupressure.

In acupressure the finger tips are used instead of needles. Though the results may not be as dramatic or as fast, they are undeniably helpful. If a contact point on the body is sore to the touch, an energy leak or congestion may be at that point, correction of which can be restored by pressure, both on the acupuncture point itself, as well as in the interior areas of the body where it relates. When congestion is eliminated, the soreness disappears and repair begins.[1]

However, bear in mind that none of the remedies I mention is claimed to *cure* anything. They merely help the body to repair itself. Doctors do not cure; it is nature, whom they may assist, that does the work.

Just because some therapies included may be new to you, it does not mean that they won't be helpful. Actually, some of them have been used for centuries, but have been suppressed because they are competitive with other treatments, or do not represent "the consensus of medical opinion." Don't be turned off by those who tell you such things are not "accepted," or are foolish. *Nothing* is foolish if it is safe (I intend to mention only safe remedies), or becomes a turning point toward some improvement, or gets even one person well. Some of these therapies have too long been kept from public view because many doctors do not believe in them. This is not surprising. For centuries the history of the medical profession is replete with examples of criticism, even persecution, of those practitioners whose treatments are not considered orthodox. One of the earlier examples of this closed-mindedness was the persecution of William Harvey, the English doctor who, in the 1600s, first discovered the circulation of the blood. Other doctors considered him a quack! Today, of course, everyone accepts circulation of the blood as of paramount importance in medicine. An example of today's resistance by orthodoxy is nutrition. Doctors are not taught nutrition in medical schools, they are taught the use of

drugs instead. Unless they have learned about it on their own—
and fortunately some have—many attack nutrition as being
worthless. Another travesty is unnecessary surgery. The body
has a hard enough time getting along with all the spare parts
with which it was born, let alone being deprived of one of them:
kidney, lung, or gall bladder, for example, merely for "experimental purposes."

Chiropractic, osteopathy and homeopathy have also been de-
nounced, yet many patients have benefitted from their use.
Homeopathy is practiced only by M.D.'s who have had the same
training as other physicians, but have merely added this new
therapy in postgraduate study after graduation from medical
school. Homeopathy is the art of using an infinitesimal amount
of a selected substance, usually natural, in a tiny inexpensive tablet which has often returned people to health within an amazingly short time, even though the disease may have existed for
years. Homeopathic substances are safe, without the dangers or
side effects of drugs. Homeopathic remedies are prescribed by a
homeopathic doctor who listens to and assesses the patient's
symptoms, in many cases without regulation medical tests or
painful exploratory surgery. Yet this system has been known to
produce healing miracles. But because there has been so much
persecution of this simple, inexpensive art, homeopathic doctors
are rare and hard to locate. If you wish to find one in your area,
see the address at the end of this chapter under references.[2]

Fortunately there is an ever-increasing group of physicians
who are beginning to use many natural remedies, including nutrition, homeopathy, even acupuncture, if allowed to by the state
in which they practice. Such open-minded doctors are getting
excellent results and are usually so popular that they are
swamped. I know several who, because they use safe, though
unusual, therapies, have had a tremendous patient recovery
rate. Due to word-of-mouth publicity by delighted patients,
others are flooding their offices. Some doctors are so busy as a
result that at intervals they are forced to close down their appointment list in order to catch up. There should be thousands
of such doctors!

If you can find one of these doctors, by all means seek his services. If not, you may have to do some self-experimenting with the same remedies they use, and which I will share with you. Is this safe on a do-it-yourself basis? Remember that you are an individual and as unique as your own fingerprints. Even a doctor cannot know, until he experiments, exactly what substances your body needs, or the potency it requires. There are, of course, some general principles which apply to everyone. Your nutritional diet represents the type of fuel you routinely put into your body to keep it running. Because the greatest cause of most illnesses today is said to be malnutrition, many people have corrected their ailments by changing their diet alone. But not everybody! Negative thinking, resulting in psychosomatic ills, unrelieved stress, and inadequate physical exercise are other important factors in health, too,

Drs. Emanuel Cheraskin and W. M. Ringsdorf, Jr. report that exercise affects every phase of body function. They present laboratory proof that daily exercise can slow down chronic disease, improve heart function, help symptoms such as uric acid levels, and even increase length of life.[3] One reason for exercise is to increase circulation to organs and glands for better performance. Another is to aid the lymph, a clear fluid which bathes every cell of the body. Lymph has no motive force such as the heart to keep it moving. It moves only when propelled by the movement of the physical body, through exercise.

The "new breed" of doctors who are very gradually becoming available are *really* beginning to put into practice the oath of Hippocrates, the father of medicine, who was concerned with natural remedies such as rest, work, eating correctly, sleeping, recreation and exercise for the patient. Twenty-five centuries ago Hippocrates recognized that much illness was psychosomatic (due to wrong thinking and faulty emotions), though the term was not used then. He also knew that doctors do not cure; that nature does the job, and that the body's goal is always aimed toward health if given a fair chance through natural approaches. Only when these measures failed did he turn to medication next, and as a final recourse, to surgery. Today the order seems to be reversed, drugs and surgery are tried first, and natural remedies—such as correct nutrition, exercise and rest—are often totally ignored.

So, if you are well enough to try some of these natural methods at home, either with or without a doctor's help, you have an advantage. There is no law (yet) which prevents your use of any remedy you wish to use, providing it is not dangerous. (Many will try to tell you that some of the methods, including vitamins, are dangerous, but you still have the final say.) Whatever you decide to do to help yourself *is your responsibility*. Your body belongs to you and is your sole property. Therefore, you can do with it as you wish. This is particularly the case because doctors consider most of the diseases discussed here to be incurable. Since this is not necessarily true, you owe it to yourself to at least give these natural remedies a try.

But since your decision is your own, you must not blame any results or lack of them on another. Different remedies work for different people. I, and the publishers, in reporting this information to you, assume no responsibility whatsoever. As long as freedom of the press exists, we can still report what help is available. It is up to you to choose it or not.

Due to my crowded schedule, I regret that I cannot answer *any* correspondence in connection with this book or supply names of doctors, products, or any other information not included. However, you will find some fascinating information for exploration on your own. Since it is safe, it is certainly worth a try. Don't you agree?

REFERENCES
(See *Bibliography* for fuller details.)

1. F. M. Houston, D.C., *The Healing Benefits of Acupressure*.
2. For names of Homeopathic doctors, write American Foundation for Homeopathy, Inc., Suite 506, 6231 Leesburg Pike, Falls Church, Virginia, 22044.
3. E. Cheraskin M.D., D.M.D., and W. M. Ringsdorf, Jr., D.M.D., M.S., *Predictive Medicine*.

2: ALCOHOLISM

A newspaper ad reads: "If you want to drink, that is your business. If you want to stop drinking, call Alcoholics Anonymous."

Undoubtedly AA is an extremely helpful organization for many excessive drinkers or alcoholics, and it deserves much credit. Twice, before his death, I heard the founder tell the moving story of how, in his own desperation, he discovered the principles of AA and passed them on to others. But this is not the *only* solution to the problem of alcoholism. There are other ways out, too, and most people, including doctors and therapists, are apparently unaware of them. Whereas the average physician considers drugs the only approach, and most psychotherapists believe that their therapy is the most successful treatment, there is still another method which is quicker, long-lasting and perhaps potentially more successful for some victims. Many alcoholics have been "cured" by this method within days, without the uncomfortable "drying out" process or the painful withdrawal symptoms. I will tell you about it and list some case histories. Meanwhile, it is unfortunate that doctors do not use this method instead of drugs, or that psychotherapists do not combine it with their therapy.

But before I tell you about this relatively unknown method, who needs such help?

Who is An Alcoholic?

How do you know when you, or a member of your family, is an alcoholic? Roger J. Williams, Ph.D., of the University of Texas, and a researcher on alcoholism for over twenty years, states that anyone who drinks enough alcohol to interfere with being a useful and productive citizen, is an alcoholic.

Women are catching up with men in overdrinking. In England the number of women alcoholics has risen from one in nine, as of a few years ago, to one in four or five, today. According to Mary Ross, director of the Council on Alcholism in Monterey, California, many women are "hidden drinkers" going on for years without their disease being suspected. Women should be made aware of early warning signals, she added, and cited the drinking of liquor to relieve depression and calm nerves as indications of alcohol being used as a drug. Other danger signals are:

—The ability to hold liquor well.
—An increasing irritability when drunk.
—A steady increase in the amount of drink.
—Actual intoxication occurring more frequently.
—Lying about the number of drinks—minimizing them.
—Taking morning drinks—or drinks upon waking up.
—Missing work or household duties.
—Neglecting children

An extremely common trait of women alcoholics, according to Mrs. Ross, is the hiding of liquor. "There could be a handy bottle of sherry in with the potatoes. One woman I know who has a swimming pool filled her chlorine bottles with vodka."

One of the most startling findings of the results of alcoholism in women is that babies born to alcoholics were, themselves, alcoholics.

Dr. David Abramson, director of the intensive care unit at Georgetown University Hospital, Maryland, found that the babies were afflicted with the early stages of liver disease and actually went through the symptoms of alcohol withdrawal for the one or two weeks necessary to wean them from alcohol. Mothers of three infants Dr. Abramson treated admitted taking from four to five cocktails per night to something less than a fifth per day.

Doctors in other parts of the country have observed in babies of alcoholic mothers withdrawal symptoms such as nervousness, crankiness and tremors, which continued well after birth and were not considered temporary. Dr. David W. Smith of Seattle, one of the first physicians to do such research, stated; "There was actually alcohol on one baby's breath . . . the alcohol gets to the fetus as it gets to the mother." (*San Francisco Chronicle*, Feb. 27, 1975.)

Meanwhile, at this writing, in New York State, alcoholics of both sexes are increasing at the rate of 20,000 per year. California alone has one million or more alcoholics. And in San Francisco there are an estimated 145,000 alcoholics, according to the National Council on Alcoholism. This city is vying with Washington D.C. and Miami, Fla. for the national alcoholic title. Alcohol is now considered the most used and abused *drug*, and alcoholism the third greatest health problem, following heart disease and cancer. The University of California Medical Center estimates that more than 90% of American adults rely on alcohol as a favorite "drug."

The trouble is that many drinkers, considered alcoholics by their friends or families, will not admit it to themselves, thus they resist treatment, the need for which becomes progressive. And the longer one waits, the harder it is to turn back, in many cases. Dr. Roger J. Williams writes: "The alcohol-prone individuals are in a sense marked men or women for life. They never are wholly out of danger as far as affliction is concerned and must 'watch their step' continually as long as they live."

There are others who can take a drink or leave it without becoming compulsive drinkers; and there are those for whom alcohol has little or no attraction. Alcoholic beverages just do not interest them. They do not like the taste or the effect. There is also a vast difference between wanting a drink and *needing* a drink. Many people can stop after one drink, whereas the alcoholic, even after long periods of abstinence, can take one drink and be off again on the nonstop drinking route. Dr. Williams considers this compulsion the common denominator of alcoholics. He says, "An alcoholism-prone individual, especially a severe case, in unable to stop of his own volition. Once he has started, each drink calls for another."

Dr. Melvin E. Page D.D.S., of the Page Foundation, St. Petersburg, Florida, a specialist in biochemistry and endocrinology, believes that a well or healthy man cannot drink without experiencing physical problems. Thus he classifies alcoholism as an illness, and warns that anyone who *needs* a drink should look suspiciously to his state of health.

Why Do People Begin Drinking?

Before choosing a successful treatment to reverse alcoholism, it is important to understand why a person became a compulsive drinker in the first place. It is apparently true that heredity may be a factor in some cases, but this is an exception. Usually the cause of drinking is psychological, or physiological, or both; or it can start with a psychological cause and end up with a physiological result. Let's look at the psychological causes first.

Some people start drinking because of social pressure. A teenager may drink experimentally because his parents do, or because his friends, whom he admires, encourage him to. Once he starts, he becomes hooked. But adults do the same thing. They may start drinking at the inevitable cocktail party because everyone else is drinking. Or they may feel insecure, unsuccessful in some way, and ape those whom they admire, hoping some of their sophistication will rub off on them. Alcohol, like sugar and tobacco, is habit forming. The more you have, the more you want. The reverse is also true: the less you have, the less you want. For the average person, *not* the alcoholic, it is possible to re-educate and reverse such a craving by oneself.

But there are other psychological causes for drinking. The victim may be tired, frightened, depressed or worried; lonely or unsuccessful in some area of his or her life, or unhappy; he may feel unloved, misunderstood, rejected, or taken advantage of. He may take a drink to give him courage or confidence to make a decision, a speech, or to try to face a problem. If he is unpopular, a drink may make him feel accepted. Or he may drink to compensate for sexual, financial or family failure; to pep himself up, quiet himself down, or to get to sleep. He may feel unworthy, fearful and insecure, sorry for himself, or drink to get himself through a day, or at the end of a day to reward himself for getting through it. He may drink to soften criticism, failure, or boredom. In other words, he uses alcohol as an *anesthetic*. Since many alcoholics are emotionally immature and are trying to cover up their weaknesses from themselves (and, they hope, from others), the euphoric effect of alcohol is the only way they know to live with themselves and their problems. And the longer the addiction continues, the less able they are to face and handle their problems realistically. Therapy can certainly help such people *before* they become addicts.

The average alcoholic is also a lonely person, basically. He thrives on companionship. But later he resents those (friends and family) who want to help him. He becomes antisocial and resentful of any interference. Those who live alone may finally go into hiding with their only solace, the bottle.

Prevention of Alcoholism

Prevention of alcoholism is easier than cure. Once the brain begins to be affected along with other organs of the body, stability, will power and resistance are progressively weakened. Therapy is certainly indicated early in the game, but so is the elimination of alcohol itself. This was proved in the case of children, who are particularly susceptible, when in the 1930s the French government gave wine to school children as a digestive aid. This resulted in tens of thousands of children as young as six years old becoming addicted.

Since you will soon see that alcohol is related to nutrition (it washes the B vitamins and magnesium out of the body, as well as displacing health-building foods), it becomes obvious that alcohol can interfere with the health, both present and future, of children and adults alike. It can act as a poison to many. As Dr. Williams says, the best way to prevent a fire is to stop it before it starts, i.e., to prevent alcoholism, don't drink!

The Nutritional Method of Reversing Alcoholism

Nutrition has proved to be a surprisingly good weapon against alcoholism, a far more successful and safer approach than drugs. Dr. Williams, who is the world-renowned director of the Clayton Foundation Biochemical Institute, University of Texas, has done research on alcoholism from a nutritional point of view for many years, so this is not a new idea. Dr. Williams is noted for his work with the B vitamin, pantothenic acid, and for his pioneer work with another B vitamin, folic acid; yet for some reason his work with alcoholism has had little publicity. He learned some surprising facts about alcohol in tests with laboratory rats. He found that those animals which were poorly nourished craved more alcohol, *but lost their craving when given certain nutrients in which they were found to be deficient.* Dr. Williams says, "This observation has been confirmed hundreds of times in many laboratories so there is no question about it."

For those who insist that the cause of alcoholism is psychological only, Dr. Williams has a startling answer. He says, "I have encountered too many severe alcoholics who had happy homes, who were happy in their work, and appeared to be less in need of escape than most, and yet they were alcoholics." He found that in people, as well as in laboratory animals who were alcohol-prone, there can be, due to disturbed cellular metabolism, a "physiological craving induced as a physiological agent . . . and without it, typical alcoholism would not exist." This physiological derangement occurs in the hypothalamus (a portion of the brain related to appetite control) and, according to Dr. Williams, the hypothalamus becomes mildly poisoned by the alcohol, which makes the so-called "body wisdom," or appetite guide, unreliable, leading to abnormal craving for alcohol and the explanation for one drink leading to another. This distortion of "body wisdom" is recognized in other habit-forming tastes: a craving for candy (sugar) and tobacco. Many who start eating sweets can't stop, and one cigarette leads to another. Thus, concludes Dr. Williams, after many years of research, alcoholism is not limited to psychological causes, but has a definitely physiological cause in many instances.

It is good news that, like the laboratory animals, the craving need not continue unabated. If the alcoholic is supplied with certain nutrients missing from his body, the craving can be halted and even reversed. I recall Dr. Williams telling of a graduate chemistry student who was about to give up just when his graduate degree was in sight, because of his terrible craving for alcohol, which was interfering with his work. The student reluctantly decided to swallow his pride, and ask Dr. Williams for help. When he also swallowed the missing nutrients that should have been in his diet as a protection against alcohol-proneness, his craving subsided and he earned his degree with no further trouble.

In this case, however, the man had to *seek* help; not every alcoholic will lift a finger to help himself. It may take a shock—and a big one—to bring him to this point. For this reason, I will list the disturbances caused by alcohol. Perhaps a glance at this list will provide the necessary impetus to seek help, before it is too late, through a simple, painless and surprisingly quick nutritional treatment.

Physical Results of Alcoholism
—Brain disturbance, temporary at first, later becoming chronic. (Brains of alcoholics studied after death by medical students have been found too mushy and disintegrated for dissection.)

—Blackouts, complete loss of memory, hypoglycemia, physical illness, headache, indigestion.

—Mental disease.

—Weight gain from edema (body water storage).

—Extreme nervousness, rages, irritability, tremors.

—Serious liver damage from which many alcoholics have died.

—Degeneration of heart tissue.

—Visual defects.

—Aggravation of schizophrenia and epilepsy.

—Elevation of blood cholesterol.

—Aggravation of high blood pressure, bronchitis, diabetes.

—Alcohol is involved in 50 percent of American traffic accidents, resulting in 25,000 fatalities each year. It also leads to arrest in 2½ million nontraffic offenses.

—Reduces life expectancy ten to twelve years.

Am I an Alcoholic?

A "yes" answer to three or more of the following questions compiled by the National Council on Alcoholism indicates a definite drinking problem.

Do you:

1. Require a drink the next morning?
2. Prefer (or like) to drink alone?
3. Lose time from work due to drinking?
4. Crave a drink at a definite time daily?
5. Get the inner shakes if you don't drink?
6. Drink to obtain social ease?
7. Drink for self-encouragement or to relieve marked feelings of inadequacy?
8. Suffer from complete loss of memory while or after drinking (blackouts)?

Since drinking, have you:

9. Become careless of your family's welfare?
10. Become irritable?
11. Thought less of your husband or wife?

12. Had difficulty in sleeping?
13. Become more impulsive?
14. Had less self-control?
15. Felt decreased initiative?
16. Felt decreased ambition?
17. Felt that your sexual potency has suffered?
18. Shown marked dislikes and hatreds?
19. Turned to an inferior environment?
20. Displayed increased jealousy?

Is drinking:
21. Harming your family in any way?
22. Changing your personality?
23. Causing you bodily complaints?
24. Decreasing your efficiency?
25. Making you harder to get along with?
26. Endangering your health?
27. Affecting your peace of mind?
28. Jeopardizing your business?
29. Clouding your reputation?

Nutritional Treatment for Alcoholics

According to Dr. Emanuel Cheraskin, a highly respected professor at the University of Alabama, no one who follows good nutritional practices ever becomes an alcoholic. This has been proved by studies with rats, under the supervision of Dr. Roger J. Williams at the University of Texas, and was duplicated at Loma Linda University in California.

The specific nutrients used by Dr. Williams in his rehabilitating program with alcohol-prone animals have been incorporated in a vitamin/mineral supplement for alcohol-prone human beings. Dr. Williams has given this formula, gratis, for the benefit of the public. He derives no income from the product, regardless of who sells it. These supplements are sold under various trade names.[1] The formula is as follows:

Vitamins
Vitamin A: 20,000 I.U.
Vitamin D: 1,000 I.U.
Vitamin C (ascorbic acid):   200 mg.
B vitamins
  thiamin (B-1):   4 mg.
  riboflavin (B-2)   4 mg.
  pyridoxin (B-6):   6 mg.
  niacinamide (B-3):   40 mg.
  pantothenate: 40 mg.
  B-12:   10 mcg.
  inositol: 200 mg.
  choline: 200 mg.
Vitamin E (tocopherol):   200 mg.

Minerals
Calcium: 300 mg.
Phosphate: 250 mg.
Magnesium: 100 mg.
Copper: 1 mg.
Iodine: 0.1 mg.
Iron: 10 mg.
Manganese: 1 mg.
Zinc: 5 mg.

There are numerous case histories revealing the success of treatment with this vitamin/mineral supplement. These are included in Dr. Williams' book, *Alcoholism, the Nutritional Approach,* a small but wonderful book[2] which, in my opinion, should be owned by every alcoholic, or family of an alcoholic. There are many convincing testimonials cited in the book:

—One man, after taking the capsules for approximately a month, stated that he no longer had a craving for whiskey.

—A wife wrote that, after five years, her husband was still free of his compulsive drinking.

—Another wife, who admitted that she had been spiking her husband's breakfast tomato juice secretly with these vitamins and minerals, reported the good results as follows: "I would never have believed that vitamins could have helped my husband who has been a periodic drinker for twenty years."

A final testimony was written by yet another wife after sixteen months of use of the vitamin/mineral supplement: "My husband had been drinking about 26 oż. of whiskey a day for about 10 years . . . and had tried AA without success. He tried the supplement with immediate success. Within a couple of months he was completely cured and hasn't had a single relapse."

Has everyone been helped? Dr. Williams has no definite method of follow-up, but of two dozen patients who reported in after reading the book, and taking the supplements, 50% were greatly benefitted. A large percentage remained free of symptoms as long as they also practiced the following added dietary recommendations:

Nutritional Diet to be Used with the Vitamin/Mineral Supplement

1. Plenty of good protein: poultry, meat, fish, eggs, cheese and milk.
2. Some fresh fruit, preferably raw.
3. Some green and yellow vegetables, raw and cooked.
4. Unsaturated oils for salad dressings.
5. Avoidance of refined and processed food and man-made carbohydrates such as starchy, sugary foods. Such foods are devoid of natural minerals and vitamins.
6. Plenty of rest.
7. Regular indoor and outdoor exercise. This helps circulation to the hypothalamus, the appetite center of the brain.

Dr. Williams mentions one other nutrient,[3] a harmless nutritional protein substance, or amino acid, called glutamine (not to be confused with glutamic acid). This is not readily available but can be procured. Dr. Williams suggests that alcoholics take two grams daily. He reports that it has been used on human alcoholics with benefit, and tells of one dramatic case in which an alcoholic of long standing stopped drinking spontaneously on taking the glutamine. He experienced no disturbance from the treatment and was not even aware that it was being added to his drinking water, as a result of a physician's prescription.

The type of treatment for alcoholics must be chosen according to individual needs. Whereas all experts are in agreement that an alcoholic should practice total abstinence, this can be achieved by different routes. Nutrition may be the easiest, and can be provided quietly, even secretly, by family members, should the person concerned refuse help. Those who submit to therapy will no doubt benefit from this approach as well. However, many people are afraid of psychiatrists or other therapists, and others are turned off by the religious element in AA. The decision should be left to the alcoholic and his family after weighing the pros and cons of all approaches.

Is There Any Benefit in Alcohol?

Is alcohol always dangerous? The answer to this question lies in the individual. If he has a physiological derangement and is alcohol-prone, the answer could well be *yes*, it is dangerous for him. However, if he is one who can take a drink or leave it, perhaps he is safe. We have all read of oldsters who have had a small snifter daily and lived to a ripe old age, so we dare not generalize. *Each person is different.* It has been estimated that one in twenty individuals becomes addicted to alcohol.

Some physicians believe wine is safer than tranquilizers when taken at the end of a hard day, and many doctors prescribe a glass of dinner wine for hospital patients, as well as for the elderly who have nothing else to look forward to. If the person's body chemistry is not out of balance, and he takes no more than 3 oz. of wine close to, or with, his meal, this may be acceptable *for that person.* More than this amount of wine could easily lead to addiction, however. "Winos" are not uncommon.

A report (*Organic Consumer Report*, July 12, 1966) stated that the instant aging of wine is now being made possible in this country by a process devised at a West Coast university. The wine is said to be bombarded with ultrasonic waves and irradiated with cobalt-60, an atomic ray. The time may well have arrived when wine should carry a list of ingredients and methods of processing on labels to protect those who drink it.

What does a controlled alcoholic, or a nondrinker, do at a cocktail party? Most hostesses today can provide substitutes such as: tomato juice, milk, fruit juice, bouillion (on the rocks), or various nonalcoholic mixes. Try to avoid the cola drinks and others containing sugar.

REFERENCES
(See *Bibliography* for fuller details.)

1. "Nutricol Forte." Write for prices to Vitamin-Quota, 1125 Crenshaw Blvd., Los Angeles, Ca. 90019, or "G-154 Nutrins," General Nutrition Corp., 418 Weed St., Pittsburgh, Pa. 15222.
2. Roger J. Williams, Ph.D., *Alcoholism, the Nutritional Approach*.
3. Write for information on glutamine to Erex Health products, P.O. Box 278, Barnhart, Mo. 63012.

3: ALLERGIES

There are various types of disturbing substances in today's environment which can cause mild to violent reactions in many people. Although these reactions are all loosely lumped as allergies, they may range from true allergies, through intolerances of certain foods and substances, to reactions resulting from pollution.

There are methods of outwitting many of these allergic disturbances. First, the sources must be identified—a difficult but not always an impossible task. Second, once discovered, they should be avoided if possible. Third, and most important, general health and resistance should be built up so that an immunity to them can be established.

What causes allergies?

Certain substances which disturb some hypersensitive people are known as allergens. They may cause allergies in these people, but not in others. Hay fever, for example, can be caused by airborne substances and/or direct contact with pollens, fur or feathers of pets (even feathers in a pillow). As an example, a seven-year-old girl was found one morning lying on her bed in a pool of blood, due to a nosebleed. This happened again and again while doctors frantically looked for the cause. Eventually it was discovered: an allergy to the pillow on which the child slept. When a pillow of a different filling was substituted, the bleeding stopped.

Two years later, the family was visiting a relative in another city, and the child was assigned to a room of her own. On awakening her in the morning, the mother again found her child surrounded with blood. A change in pillows promptly stopped the bleeding during the remainder of their visit. House dust is a common offender; it can lurk in window shades or rugs, as well as on a piano. Mold is another offender. A man who had suffered for ten years from small itching blisters on the palms of his hands and on his feet, was tested by an allergist who found that he was allergic to mold. But the man insisted there was no mold in his house or place of work. Later, when he was rebuilding his house, erected on a wooden foundation upon a damp piece of ground, he found the wooden foundation to be riddled with mold. When he substituted a concrete foundation, his eczema disappeared.

Other allergies can come from fumes from appliances: gas stoves, heaters, furnaces, even though a leak is not noticeable; *any* aerosol spray, since it is gas-propelled, becomes an added hazard to the contents, such as paint, lacquer, room deodorant, hair spray or oven cleaners. One woman, who nearly collapsed while her head was inside her oven as she used her spray oven cleaner, was rushed to the hospital by ambulance just in time to save her life. Most chemicals which smell are also suspect: floor cleaners, waxes, cleaning fluids, chlorine bleaches in cleansers, toilet bowl cleaners (a combination of some of these household cleaners has proved fatal due to producing toxic gases), as well as odorless insecticides in spray cans, or even in wallpaper and carpets. Cosmetics, perfumes, soaps, dentrifices, and *in*organic hair dyes have caused widespread trouble. A woman who has tell-tale bags, or dark circles, under her eyes may rightly suspect poisoning from *in*organic hair dyes. (There are safe, organic alternatives explained in my book, *Secrets of Health and Beauty*).[1]

Smoking, even by others, has actually made adults and children ill without anyone suspecting the cause.

Plastics are also attracting attention, particularly those that smell, and some that don't. The FDA is questioning liquor in plastic bottles, and the FTC is warning about plastic dishes and coffee cups, such as those found on planes. Many ordinary fabrics are also suspect. A woman who "itched" in the winter, but not in the summer, discovered she was allergic to wool clothing. Some people are even allergic to wool carpeting, although it might be due to the insecticide or moth proofing commercially impregnated in the fiber. Certain synthetic fibers irritate some people.

Drugs are common disturbers, including antibiotics, tranquilizers and many others. Even some vitamins cause trouble for some people, though this is often due to the sugar or chocolate or other coating on the tablets or capsules. For this reason, a few reputable supplement companies are dispensing with tablet coatings.

In the food department the list is endless. If you have trouble locating your allergy, as one expert suggests, eliminate milk, chocolate and cola drinks first, for a week or so. If you do not feel dramatically better, try wheat next.

However, there are other culprits, harder to pinpoint. Claude A. Frazier, M.D., of Asheville, North Carolina, states, "I, and, I suspect, a goodly number of my colleagues in other medical specialties, especially general practitioners, are deeply concerned about the role both additives and refinements are playing in our nation's rising incidence of degenerative disease and our relatively poor health generally . . . I believe that additives, both intentional and unintentional, that turn up in our food products in astonishing quantity and variety are responsible for a good part of the rise in allergy diseases in our population."

The way out of this dilemma is, of course, to eat food in its natural state instead of that which is tampered with and commonly available in our grocery stores. Not only is the trouble in the foods themselves, but in what is done to them. They are sprayed, gassed, colored, preserved for longer shelf life and generally perverted. At least 3,200 additives, at most 10,000 (by FDA figures), are present in our foods.

Although these additives occur in countless foods, some listed on the labels, some not, few people realize the serious allergic reactions which can result. For example, Stephen D. Lockey, Sr., M.D., F.A.C.A., Emeritus Chief, Department of Allergy, Lancaster General Hospital, Lancaster, Pennsylvania, cites several average cases. Writing in *Consumers' Research Magazine* (Washington, N.J. 07882) May, 1974, he tells of a member of a physician's own family who suffered from sudden weakness, extreme fatigue, and swelling at the back of the tongue. The reactions were traced to the eating of corn flakes or instant potatoes, both of which contain the common preservatives, BHA and BHT.

At this writing, there is almost no dry cereal which does not contain these preservatives. Read your labels! In addition to additives in the food, there are other hazards. Foods are stored in tin cans (the tin affects some people); they are cooked in aluminum cooking ware. They are grown in insecticide-contaminated soil or sprayed with fungicides or other poisons. It is a wonder that we get along as well as we do.

As to foods *per se*, some reactions to them may be due to allergy; others to intolerances. The difference is that an allergen may exist in the *food*. In an intolerance, the trouble may lie in the *person*. For example, some people are allergic to milk because, after weaning, they did not continue milk drinking. As a result, an enzyme, lactase, needed to digest the milk sugar, lactose, is no longer functioning in their bodies. So this is the fault of the person, not the food. (Black people as a group tend to be allergic to milk.) On the other hand, allergy to chocolate, which one well-known medical clinic classifies as a No. 1 allergy because it is so common in so many people, *may* be explained by one or more disturbing ingredients contained in the food itself. Drug intolerance is also possible. One injection of penicillin has killed. An allergy can also result from a combination or interaction between two or more foods, or other substances.

Contaminants

There are numerous environmental contaminants accumulating in our air, water and food. These include lead, mercury, cadmium, asbestos, and various radioactive substances.[2,3] There is also smog, with its many chemical irritants, and fluoride, which is airborne as well as being deliberately placed in the water without concern for those who may be allergic to it.

We are living these days in a contaminated environment, and it is getting worse, not better.

Allergy Symptoms

If you are going to seek out a possible allergy, intolerance or contaminant (don't worry too much about which type it is), it will help you to recognize it if you know some of the possible symptoms. Let me warn you not to identify with *all* of them. It is well known that medical students develop most of the symptoms of each disease they study. Also, do not conclude prematurely that one of the symptoms explains the only cause of a chronic disturbance. These symptoms can mimic other diseases. But the reverse is also true. *Begin* with a search for an allergy. It might save you from an incorrect diagnosis of a more serious ailment, as has already happened to many people. I will cite such a case later.

All of these symptoms can be caused by, but not limited to, food allergies. For example, in one person wheat simultaneously caused unusual wakefulness at night, diarrhea, abdominal bloating, rectal itching, and depression. These symptoms disappeared when wheat was eliminated from the diet, but returned when it was continued. Wheat germ has caused a rash in one person, general lassitude and shortness of breath in another. Even wheat germ oil and Vitamin E derived from it can cause allergies for many, whereas others thrive on them.

Allergy Symptoms

Recurring headache	Gastric ulcer
Migraine	Gastric pain
Dizziness	Colitis
Irritability	Rectal itching
Nervousness	Gastrointestinal
Vague complaint of	bleeding
"not feeling well"	Asthma
Depression	Bloating
Neuralgia	Overweight
Abnormal tiredness	Underweight
Sneezing	High blood pressure
Conjunctivitis	Chest pain
Nosebleed	Heart attacks
Diabetes	Eczema
Epilepsy	Hives
Indigestion (gas,	Sinusitis
vomiting)	Stuffy and/or
Constipation	runny nose
Hemorrhoids	Rapid pulse
Diarrhea	(tachycardia)
Heartburn	Shortness of breath
Abdominal pain	Hay fever
Gall bladder pain	Face and eye swelling

The same food can also cause different symptoms in different people. Fresh or frozen orange juice produced a rash in one woman; diarrhea, rectal itching, nosebleed and high blood pressure in another.

Many allergies are multiple and may be caused by multiple allergens. One man suffered from heartburn, indigestion, 3-day migraines and face swelling. An allergist found his allergens were wheat, sugar and coffee. When all these foods were eliminated, his health returned.

A 70-year-old woman suffered from physical tiredness, constipation and overweight, plus a susceptibility to colds, devastating tiredness and shifting neuralgia. She had lived with these problems for thirty years! An allergist identified her allergens as milk, oranges, peanuts, lemons, carrots, beets, asparagus and onions. On avoiding these foods, her symptoms soon disappeared; she happily lost thirty-five pounds, and has remained well ever since.

The late Arthur F. Coca, M.D., allergy specialist, found a woman patient who was allergic to fifteen foods, five of which, including sugar, she was unable to eat at all. The other ten she could eat once a week with no trouble. Her symptoms disappeared and her health became perfect when she followed a strict regimen.

Another allergy specialist, Granville F. Knight, M.D., reports the case of a woman with an eruption on her back, frequent urination, itching and congested eyes, overall fatigue, nasal obstruction and sneezing. She obtained relief when her allergens, milk and dairy products, house dust and pollens were discovered and eliminated. Another of Dr. Knight's patients suffered from asthma in childhood; had a nervous breakdown after childbirth, and displayed nervousness, dizziness and fatigue. Diagnosis by other doctors had been "neuroses" (the troubles were supposedly all in her mind). Yet, when Dr. Knight identified her allergens as beef, commercial bread, citrus fruits, lamb, rice, potato, banana, chocolate, egg and cinnamon, and the patient eliminated these foods, her health improved to the point that life became worth living once more and she was no longer considered "neurotic."[4]

Pinpointing Your Allergies

Locating your allergy, or allergies (since they usually come in groups) is not easy. In times past, allergists subjected patients to skin tests, pricking the skin with a number of known allergens. Today the number of disturbers has reached the thousands, often baffling patient and doctor alike. Skin tests are now usually limited to those causing hay fever, asthma, or similar reactions. This would include certain pollens, molds, household dust, and dander from dogs, cats and rabbits. The skin tests have very little value in determining food allergies, and none at all for chemicals, according to Dr. Knight. Patch tests are used to help determine causes of eczema, skin rashes, poison oak and ivy, and certain allergies to chemicals. But chemicals are proliferating so rapidly that no one can keep up with them.

For example, one allergen which has been little suspected finally came to light after two years of searching by a friend of mine. She was suffering from a rapid pulse. Tests by two doctors—a heart specialist and a general practitioner—revealed no heart trouble and no known cause. Quite accidentally, to my surprise, *I* found it! My friend lived in a distant city and had invited me to spend the weekend at her house. She politely gave up her own bedroom, with connecting bath, and moved into a less convenient room. When I walked into her own bedroom, I was nearly overwhelmed by the odor of mothballs! I opened her closet door and the fumes all but asphyxiated me. That night I opened wide every window in the room, but still the fumes were overwhelming. The next morning I told my friend about an article I had read, "Beware of Those Mothballs," written by Francis Silver, ecologist.[5] As a result, my friend threw out the mothballs and her fast pulse disappeared. Strangely, even though the odor had almost asphyxiated me, she no longer noticed it. This is because the sense of smell becomes fatigued, as every woman knows who sniffs many perfumes before buying one. Smokers also tend to lose their keen sense of smell. So a housewife can become unaware of the many odors of the products she uses.

The real tragedy today lies not only in the home, but in the school. Your children are subjected to an unbelievable array of chemicals. They may develop headaches, listlessness, unexplained fatigue and many other symptoms without anyone guessing the cause. Even personality disorders, as well as physical problems and poor grades, can result. One couple, who became concerned about pollutants disturbing their children, first began at home—where they did not need permission—to remove many offenders which produce chemical fumes. They removed every possibility including faulty gas appliances, furnishings, cleaning products, cosmetics, and insecticides. Next they decided to investigate the impure air in their local schools.

This search turned into a dramatic project! Mrs. Kathleen A. Blume, and another mother, Mrs. June Larson, received permission from the school board, and assistance from Theron G. Randoph, M.D., internationally known ecological allergy expert of Chicago, and Francis Silver, already mentioned in connection with the mothballs. These enterprising women invaded the school's supply-storage closets, janitor supplies, locker rooms, rest-rooms, cafeterias, kitchens and classrooms, sniffing their way through both on weekdays and Saturdays. At times the stench was so great they had to step outdoors to clear their heads in order to continue the search. The report of their findings is published in a small paperback booklet called, *Air Pollution in the Schools* (see bibliography for details). The discoveries proved almost incredible, particularly when it was realized that the children spent an average of six hours or more a day in that school building, an environment polluted by dozens of fume-producing products. The two mothers found, for example, that janitor supplies included rest-room and toilet cleansers, bleach liquids and powders, smelly supplies for wet mopping, dry sweeping, waxing, dewaxing; furniture polish, chemically treated dust mops and dust cloths, liquid soaps and window cleaners. Most of the labels read, "DO NOT BREATHE, KEEP AWAY FROM CHILDREN." But no one had bothered to look at the labels.

But that was not all. The mothers found that school supplies for art and business and laboratory classes included dangerous substances too: aerosol sprays of insecticides, paint, enamel, lacquer, spray snow, spray plastic, solvent cleaners for business machines, room air "purifiers"; rubber cement, glues, pen markers, glass and ceramic adhesives, fixatives, stencil removers. ALL of these carried warning labels totally ignored by the adults and children who were exposed to them daily.

By the time these two women and their professional allergy advisors finished their search, safe substitutes had been found (mentioned in the Blume book) and installed. Health, scholastic and other problems improved noticeably. Of course, factories and office buildings are besieged in the same manner, providing all of this indoor pollution before a person even steps outside to inhale a deep breath of smog!

On the home front, to detect offending substances, use your nose as well as your eyes and your brain. Don't take chances and don't take anything for granted. Throw *anything* suspect away and, using rubber gloves for garden supplies, read the labels on everything. If the label carries a caution, mentions chemicals, or is printed in too-fine print to read, throw the product away before it permanently damages you or a member of your family. Watch out for insect strips in pretty containers. Children and elderly people sleeping in the same room with them have become seriously ill, and no one knew why. Such slow-release insecticides have a delayed reaction, whereas high levels kill immediately, as plane pilots who spray them onto agricultural fields can verify.

One woman with constant headaches was diagnosed as having a brain tumor, for which a doctor said brain surgery was the only solution. But she noticed that she did *not* have headaches when she visited elsewhere. Finally another doctor found the cause: garden insecticides, sprayed by her neighbor, had drifted onto her property. She sold her house, moved away, and had no more trouble. She was lucky.

Don't panic because you have become dependent upon certain instant household cleaning products. There is *one* powder cleanser that does not contain chlorine bleach. Search your supermarket shelves for it. There are other organic cleansers available, usually on a house-to-house basis, but read labels on them, too, before buying. If women have licked some problems through boycotts, they can lick others. The entire home products industry reacts to the women who use, or do not use, their products. Thus housewives can make or break them. By demanding safe substitutes, they will eventually get them if they don't give up. Meanwhile they can use what grandma used— diluted vinegar, a little household ammonia (keep windows open) and others for cleaning purposes. If you *must* use an oven cleaner, take the oven apart, put the spare parts outdoors, lay them on newspapers on the ground and, holding a thick paper towel over your nose and wearing rubber gloves on your hands, brush on the paste type of cleaner. Fumes from paste are less volatile than from sprays. Line your oven with aluminum foil to avoid spills, and perhaps you won't need to use any harsh substance at all. *Use your ingenuity!*

Finding Food Allergies

There are two ways to detect disturbing foods. The first method is the trial-and-error elimination diet. Although all ingredients may not be listed, you can save yourself much time and trouble by reading the label before you buy anything. If *any* chemicals are present in foods, avoid them! Some are new, some old, with new names. Tests of danger resulting from their use are inconclusive or usually hidden from the public. Take no chances. Let them strictly alone. This automatically eliminates many hazards—and many foods.

Keep to organic, untreated, unprocessed food as closely as possible, and you will eliminate another set of hazards such as pesticides, various sprays and other poisons. But even these, which do not show or smell, can be removed. The strawberries raised in my area are sprayed with arsenic. Until I learned how to cleanse them, I refused to touch them unless they came from my own or a neighbor's garden. Bananas are gassed, and many people who formerly thrived on them can no longer tolerate them without allergic reactions. The following method is a safe way (I use it constantly) to decontaminate them. It has been supplied by the courtesy of Hazel Parcells, Ph. D., Nutritionist, whose students swear by it.

Formula

Use ½ teaspoon of Clorox to 1 gallon of water, obtained from the usual supply. (Do not try to use any other bleach product as it will not work.)

Into this bath, place the fruits or vegetables to be treated. The thin-skinned fruits and leafy vegetables will require 10 minutes.

The root vegetables and heavy-skinned fruits will require 15 to 20 minutes. *Make a fresh bath for each group.*

Remove from Clorox bath and place into a fresh water bath for 10 to 15 minutes.

There is absolutely no aftertaste or odor of Clorox. Fruits and vegetables will all keep much longer. The wilted ones will return to a fresh crispness.

This formula has been tested for safety for ten years.

I have friends who, when they are traveling in Mexico and other countries where water may be contaminated, carry a tiny bottle of Clorox with them. Adding one drop of Clorox to a glass of water decontaminates it.

After having eliminated as many distrubing possibilities as you can, then go on a self-search to see if you experience any suspicious symptoms from foods. When the symptom appears a few hours or days after a meal, ask yourself, "What did I eat or drink recently?" Make a list of every possibility. A coworker of mine, who can take a sip of alcoholic spirits with no trouble, has definite reactions from even tiny amounts of beer or wine. Within twenty-four hours he experiences gout-like pains in his joints. Others can drink wine and beer and not spirits. It took him a while to discover the cause, but he found it.

You can start out safely with a single food, say cooked brown rice, eating as much as you wish for a day, without any added vitamins or minerals to complicate your search. A day or so on this monodiet will not hurt you and almost no one is allergic to brown rice, a nutritious food, though it does not contain Vitamin C and should not be continued too long alone for that reason. Gradually add any suspect (or nonsuspect) food; sometimes the foods you like the most will upset you the most. Wait for twenty-four hours or longer to see if any reactions appear. After establishing food allergens, then gradually add nutritional supplements, one by one. Many people test food and supplements successfully by means of a pendulum, explained in another book.[6]

Occasionally, by changing the brand or the type, you can find a food substitute that does not upset you. For example, chocolate upsets many, so try carob, which tastes similar but has not been found disturbing.

Another way to find your own allergy is by the pulse test, described fully in a book by that name.[7] Briefly stated, you take your own pulse before a meal. Then, limiting that meal to one food only, wait for half an hour after eating and take your pulse again. A slight increase is considered normal, even up to sixteen extra beats. If your pulse does not climb above eighty-four, you may be allergy-free. But if your pulse definitely quickens beyond that point, and is still high one hour after the meal, you have found your food allergy. The method is described in detail in Dr. Arthur Coca's book.

But watch for other signs too. If you suddenly start sneezing for no apparent reason, suspect that grapefruit you just ate, or the cat which jumped into your lap. You may be desensitized for reaction to cat or dog fur. According to Adelle Davis[8], a person may take 500 milligrams or more of Vitamin C (ascorbic acid) before exposure to known or suspect allergens: dog, cat and horse dander; household dust during house cleaning, or possible food disturbances, *before* going to a restaurant or party. If allergic symptoms still appear, take 500 added milligrams afterward and this will usually provide quick relief. The reason: large doses of Vitamin C act as an antihistamine, or detoxifying, agent.

If you drink milk and note severe symptoms, take action. Those who cannot tolerate regular milk usually (but not always) have no trouble with soured milks such as yogurt, kefir and acidophilus, which are necessary for calcium as well as a healthier intestinal state.

Soy milk, soy bakery products, soybeans and other soy products can cause, in *some* people, allergic reactions such as gas, diarrhea, and gastrointestinal problems. Watch out for ground meat extended with soybean meal, usually called "textured vegetable protein."

How To Overcome Your Allergies

Many allergies can be prevented or reversed. So, after a period of several months' avoidance of a food, you may gingerly try eating a tiny bit of it once or twice a week, gradually increasing the amount if no symptoms appear. But if the symptoms do return with a vengeance, don't push it. That food is not for you. A relative of mine has suffered from violent diarrhea from fresh fruit such as watermelon and cantaloupe all of her life. A friend cannot eat fresh pineapple, even though she has tried it picked ripe in Hawaii (not shipped green or over-ripe as are so many disturbing fruits available today). Such food intolerances are unique to those individuals. Tension experienced while you eat a questionable food does not help, since tension interferes with the manufacture of hydrochloric acid. This can be supplied if needed. (See *Secrets of Health and Beauty* for instructions[1]) HCL has helped some intolerances. Since hydrochloric acid usually is needed for the digestion of proteins and certain minerals, dairy products, meat, fish and poultry as well as brewer's yeast, intolerances to these foods might respond (and have in many cases) to the use of hydrochloric acid. However, fresh fruits, as mentioned above, are unique problems for some, though rarely, and perhaps are irreversible. In most cases, however, after eliminating the offending food item, symptoms often disappear within two to three days.

The best way of all to prevent or overcome allergies is to strengthen your overall physical resistance so that you will not be easy prey for every allergen that comes along. Dr. Granville F. Knight, M.D., the nutritionally-oriented allergist of Santa Monica, California, reports that "Between 60 and 90 percent of all patients coming to my office with allergic . . . complaints have shown clinical deficiency of Vitamin B complex. Diet histories in almost all cases have revealed an excessive intake of refined foods and a lack of the protective ones . . . physical degeneration and increased allergic tendencies seem to advance hand in hand." He adds that, since most deficiencies are multiple, nutrients should also be multiple.

He has reported many successful cases of allergy control by an optimum diet. Sometimes the recovery is quicker in some people than others. Dr. Knight states, "Frequently progress is slow because deficiencies have usually developed over a period of years." He stresses the use of whole, organic, unrefined food, fresh fruit and vegetables, plenty of protein—especially liver and other organ meats—whole grain cereals and breads, raw *certified* milk products, fertile eggs and vitamin/mineral supplements.[9]

Vitamin C (ascorbic acid) and particularly the bioflavonoids, have proved to be another dramatic help in allergy control. Hay fever, asthma attacks, insect bites and poison oak and ivy have yielded to massive and frequent amounts of ascorbic acid which, as previously noted, seems to act as an antihistamine and detoxifier. The amount of ascorbic acid needed varies according to the toxicity acquired.[8]

The sting of bees, wasps and hornets can be a real threat. Yellow jackets are considered the most dangerous, and up to one hundred children or adults die annually from their stings. I well remember seeing a teen-age girl, who preceded a group of us into the woods for a picnic, drop her picnic basket and return screaming, followed by a cloud of attacking yellow jackets. Only a hurried trip to a doctor, who had been alerted and was waiting for her with a hypodermic needle of adrenalin, saved her life.

If you are within reach of a doctor after being stung by yellow jackets (reactions can imitate a heart attack and be deadly), waste no time getting there for an injection of adrenalin. Some allergists believe that such hypersensitive people should always carry an adrenalin kit with them on hiking and camping trips for self-administration. However, if one is attacked for the first, or even subsequent, time, and no help is near, continued massive doses of ascorbic acid have on occasion saved lives both from insect stings and poisonous spider bites.

For prevention purposes, the entire C complex or family—known as the bioflavonoids (ascorbic acid is one factor only of this family)—are indicated, since they gradually strengthen cell permeability to help immunize the body from various allergies, especially hay fever and poison oak or ivy. By taking bioflavonoids on a regular basis and well in advance of any exposure, many people have built up an immunity to the point where their most disturbing allergy no longer bothers them.

If an emergency exposure to poison oak or ivy appears before the immunity is acquired by this method, there is a quicker approach. Some drug companies make an oral product from resins derived from poison oak or ivy. If taken several weeks before exposure, they can help to desensitize the person. Still better is a homeopathic substance called *Rhus. Tox.* (derived from poison ivy), which can be started only six days before exposure. A similar homeopathic substance named "Poison Oak tablets" is also available and works in the same manner. There may or may not be the appearance of slight symptoms of any of these immunizers. If so, they soon disappear. If the exposure comes suddenly, they may even relieve symptoms for some people. The homeopathic remedies may be found at some health stores or from any homeopathic pharmacy. If you do not find the name of such a pharmacy in your yellow pages, write for information to Standard Homeopathic Pharmacy, P.O. Box 61067, Los Angeles, California, 90061. Keep such remedies on hand for emergencies.

Often the addition of pantothenic acid (a B vitamin) brings great relief to allergy sufferers. Those who have multiple allergies may have poor adrenal gland function; liberal amounts of pantothenic acid may help cure them, although recovery may require several weeks.

An example of a natural treatment for hay fever was contributed by a reader to *Prevention* Magazine, July, 1975. The reader told of her grandfather, a chronic sufferer from hay fever, who discovered that by eating two or more 6-inch leaves of fresh comfrey a day, his hay fever was completely controlled, providing he ate the comfrey leaves throughout the season. His granddaughter, the writer of the letter, also found that her itchy eyes, drippy nose and other symptoms of hay fever responded to the use of comfrey leaves within a week. She also found that comfrey tea soothed an asthmatic, allergy-type cough both in children and adults.

Adelle Davis cites the case of a physician who remained symptom-free during exposure to house dust and pollen as long as he took pantothenic acid. Pantothenic acid should always be accompanied by the entire B complex in the form of brewer's yeast or desiccated liver, or both.[8]

Here is an exciting new allergy remedy discovered by a physician in India, Hement Pathak, M.D. He found that the use of five drops of castor oil in a little juice or water, taken on an empty stomach in the morning is often beneficial for allergies in the intestinal tract, skin and nasal passages. Dr. Pathak, an expert in Chinese medicine, discovered the antiallergic nature of castor oil used in this manner accidentally. One of his patients was highly sensitive to penicillin. Meanwhile he was being given the castor oil drops by Dr. Pathak for other purposes. Another doctor unwittingly gave this man penicillin, not knowing of his sensitivity. When the patient discovered that he had been given penicillin, he panicked, but nothing at all happened. The allergy was gone! Since then Dr. Pathak has reported 140 other cases of allergic protection by this method.

One nutritional physician who has been using this remedy finds it highly successful in his patients. You can add the five drops of castor oil to anything. If you add it to cod liver oil (mint flavored) in juice, you will never know it is there. (This remedy was reported in the *Medical Research Bulletin,* of the A.R.E. Clinic Inc., by Wm. A. McGarey, M.D., Medical Director.)

Because there is so much information about allergies which could not be included here, due to lack of space, I urge you to read the books listed in the bibliography for further help.

REFERENCES
(See *Bibliography* for fuller details.)

1. Linda Clark, *Secrets of Health and Beauty.*
2. Linda Clark, *Know Your Nutrition.*
3. Linda Clark, *Are You Radioactive? How to Protect Yourself.*

4. Granville F. Knight, M.D., F.A.C.A., "Nutritional Approach to Allergy and Infection," *Journal of Applied Nutrition*, Vol. 10, No. 3, 1957.
5. *Herald of Health*, September, 1959.
6. Linda Clark, *Get Well Naturally*.
7. Arthur F. Coca, M.D., *The Pulse Test*.
8. Adelle Davis, *Let's Get Well*.
9. Granville F. Knight, M.D., F.A.C.A., "Importance of Nutrition in Infection and Allergy," presented to the Annual Congress of the American College of Allergists, New York City, April 20, 1956.

4: ANEMIA

Many people go through life feeling not quite "with it." They envy the energy, vitality and pep of others. Although they consider themselves well, and they may not actually have any diagnosable ailment, they always feel tired, sluggish, appear pale and wan. They manage to get through the day, even through life, although it is an effort. It never occurs to them that they, too, could be energetic and vigorous, and awaken each morning with that good-to-be-alive and rarin'-to-go- feeling. Such people may be suffering from varying degrees of anemia, which in many cases can be corrected by a proper diet, or at least by some simple blood building substance or natural treatment. This, in turn, can make life worth living once more.

I knew one woman who dragged around for five long years wondering if she would ever feel well and strong again. She "tried everything," hoping that her energy would return during the day and that she would not fall into bed at seven o'clock every evening exhausted. Various practitioners had found nothing seriously wrong with her and had about convinced her that her trouble was imaginary or psychosomatic. Finally, the pallor of her skin and nails provided the clue to her own discovery that she was anemic. Her condition was borderline, often called secondary or nutritional anemia. When she stepped up the intake of certain natural substances, her vitality returned and her problem was solved. She now feels like a new person.

There are various types of anemia, but according to government statistics, the majority of people suffer from a simple type only. Other more complex types are diagnosable and treatable only by physicians. A blood test by a doctor can confirm a true or more serious type of anemia. Although the medical diagnosis of simple anemia is quicker and more specific, if you wish to diagnose and treat your own simple anemia, you must first know what it is all about.

Symptoms of Anemia

If you are anemic, you run the risk of not only feeling half alive, but also failing to realize your full potential of good looks. Even a prolonged, slight anemia can ruin your appearance, changing your facial expression from a happy, alive one into a haggard one, with lines of strain, premature wrinkles, and a gray, pasty skin color. Your eyes can become dull and tired looking, too. And your hair can turn prematurely gray or be lacklustre. Even your body droops.

Other symptoms include: poor memory, fuzzy thinking, weakness, dizziness, fatigue, lack of energy and endurance, shortness of breath on exertion, wounds that heal slowly, headaches, loss of libido in men, mental depression, pale fingernails (often with vertical ridges), paleness, or a gray or slightly yellow skin color, pale lips, ear lobes and mucous membrane. (Draw down your lower eyelid. If you are anemic, the mucous membrane will appear whitish-pink instead of a vibrant, healthy color.)

What is Anemia?

Anemia, which literally means "lacking in blood," is a shortage of a good quality or quantity or rich red blood cells and coloring matter. People who are unaware of this condition believe that their symptoms, which they do not understand, are fate, and that they will have to live with them forever. This is not so.

Every day, approximately 1,000,000,000,000 (one trillion) new blood cells must be manufactured by your body. If there is not enough iron in your blood, it cannot carry oxygen to the cells to enable them to breathe, throw off waste products or replace old cells with new ones. Red cells live approximately 120 days, are being destroyed and replaced daily. The red coloring matter is called hemoglobin. There are several blood testing scales. According to one, each person should have 100 percent of hemoglobin (or about 15 grams) to 100 cc (½ cup) of blood, and a blood count of 5 million red cells per millimeter. On this scale, anemia exists when the hemoglobin is less than 80 percent. A usual high average ranges from 80-95. If your hemoglobin is 70-85, you may have borderline anemia; if it is below 60, you have true anemia; and at 35, transfusions are given. Dr. H. E. Judy reported to an American Medical Association clinical meeting that in a study of 7,000 women, though the standard hemoglobin for women is about 95, the average woman tested only about 86, largely due to loss of blood through the menstrual cycle.[1]

Causes of Anemia

Because of TV commercials which stress "tired blood" and the need for iron, most people think that in addition to menstrual loss in women, a lack of iron is the *only* cause of anemia. Not true. Iron may be a factor in many, even most, cases of anemia, but this does not mean that a person, or even a doctor, should consider using questionable iron remedies for the condition. In the first place, if the person is not anemic (continuous fatigue can also be due to other causes), the result may be dangerous as you will soon see. Even if one *is* anemic, the wrong type of iron can still be dangerous.

There is actually no shortage of iron in the American diet, *if the foods eaten are not refined.* Thus a person living largely on refined foods can easily shortchange himself on iron, although there is a plentiful supply which is free for the eating.

However, even on an excellent diet, some people cannot use the iron they eat. The reason: they lack sufficient digestive acid, known as hydrochloric acid, *and acid is needed to digest iron so that it can be assimilated,* and be put to use in the body.

Dr. E. Hugh Tuckey, formerly of San Francisco, now retired, is one of the few practitioners who has done research in depth on hydrochloric acid (usually abbreviated as HCL). Some people cringe when they hear the word "acid," due to being hypnotized by TV commercials into believing they have too much acid; so they immediately resort to taking antacids. Dr. Tuckey considers this pure folly. After studying hundreds of patients, he learned that the symptoms of *too little* acid mimic the symptoms of *too much* acid, and that more people suffer from the effects of too little than from too much. He has reversed numerous cases of indigestion and excessive gas by prescribing HCL tablets. Drs. E. Cheraskin and W. M. Ringsdorf, Jr. agree. They report that in one study of 3,484 persons selected because of their complaints of gastroinestinal distress, 27 percent were found to have little or no stomach acid, with an increasing frequency among the aging.[2]

After trying many types, Dr. Tuckey prescribed tablets of hydrochloric acid-betaine-with-pepsin with great success. The dosage and full directions for using this natural digestive supplement are explained in my book, *Secrets of Health and Beauty,*[3] which I will not repeat here, due to lack of space. Both the tablets and the book, in paperback edition, are available at health stores.

However, if for some reason HCL is not available, apple cider vinegar, though less effective than HCL according to Dr. Tuckey, can pinch-hit. Dr. D. C. Jarvis in his book, *Folk Medicine,* has stated that animals given vinegar, showed an improvement in hemoglobin, as proved on autopsy. He writes, "Turning to human beings, it is true that vinegar with water at each meal increases the amount of hemoglobin in the blood, which means that more red blood cells carrying hemoglibin are present."[4]

Anemia may also result from lack of protein. To raise the hemoglobin even 10 points, 80 grams or 3 oz. of protein are necessary. But some people cannot assimilate protein. So again, hydrochloric acid comes to the rescue and helps digest it (as well as iron and calcium), thus eliminating gas and other gastrointestinal distress resulting from undigested protein. Anemia can also result from stress, since stress can interfere with the body's manufacture of hydrochloric acid. So the chain reaction becomes complete, with HCL playing the star role.

There is still another little-known cause of anemia, intestinal parasites or worms. These are more common than supposed. Hookworm (common in the southeastern United States), pinworms, round worms and tapeworms feed on the host's (yours) supply of blood as well as on the vitamins that you need. Twenty-five hookworms can consume half an ounce of blood every twenty-four hours.[5] A tapeworm has been found to cause a shortage of Vitamin B-12, a deficiency which in turn can cause anemia. Garlic, raw, or in perle form (at health stores) can help vanquish some types of intestional parasites. There are also herbal remedies said to remove these parasites.[6] For explanation of how parasites are acquired, see my book, *Get Well Naturally* (paperback edition at health stores) p.162-4. Continous dark undereye circles, grinding the teeth during sleep, or a continuously itching nose may be indications of parasites.

Vegetarianism can also be a definite cause of anemia. Don't underestimate the great importance of protein in this ailment. Vitamin B-12, which is usually found in animal protein, is a *must* for preventing or correcting simple or serious types of anemia. Prevention is much easier than cure for a deficiency of B-12. Once serious manifestations of its lack have occurred, it is *not* a do-it-yourself treatment.

B-12 is not only difficult to get in food, it is difficult to assimilate by mouth. This is why, in serious conditions, doctors resort to injections.

B-12 occurs in microscopic amounts in foods. Animal protein is almost the only source where it occurs naturally in sufficient, necessary amounts. Liver is the best source; kidney, muscle meats, fish and dairy products (milk, eggs and cheese) are also good sources. It is found in *traces* only in some other foods, especially in vegetables, a negligible source. Peanuts, seaweed and Concord grapes, and also soybeans contain some B-12, although raw soybean flour is deficient in B-12 and creates a need for more of this Vitamin. Wheat germ contains some B-12, and brewer's yeast only if the yeast is bred specifically to include it. B-12 has been found in mouldy cheese, such as roquefort, and has been found to increase 15 percent during a three-month cheese-ripening process. A few plants including comfrey contain a small amount of it, but not enough to correct a deficiency. Desiccated liver, as well as fresh liver, are perhaps the most dependable sources of B-12.

In her book, *Let's Get Well*, Adelle Davis says: "Vegetarians are particulary subject to pernicious anemia unless they eat generous amounts of milk (products) and eggs . . . people who have followed a vegetarian diet without milk or eggs for five years or longer often develop sore mouths and tongues, menstrual disturbances and a variety of nervous symptoms including a 'needles and pins' feeling in hands and feet, neuritis, pain and stiffness in the spine and difficulty in walking. All of these symptoms, which are danger signals, dramatically clear up provided Vitamin B-12 is obtained."[7]

This warning explains why Carlton Fredericks, Ph.D., and other nutritionists urge people to eat some animal protein (or dairy product) with each meal.

Even this precaution may not insure protection once serious symptoms have set in. Vitamin B-12-deficient people lack one or more substances in the stomach for its absorption. There has long existed a belief that an "intrinsic factor" derived from animal stomach is a must for those afflicted with pernicious anemia. Without it, the vitamin has appeared to be ineffectual. Although the belief still persists, "intrinsic factor" is now available by prescription only.

Miss Davis writes: "Provided iron and Vitamin C are obtained with hydrochloric acid, they stimulate the production of the body's intrinsic factor sufficiently so that persons with mild pernicious anemia can take smaller doses."

She adds: "If individuals with pernicious anemia who take hydrochloric acid with each meal to assure the absorption of nutrients were to adhere to a completely adequate diet . . . the reverse (of symptoms) could probably be shown."

And Miss Davis warns: "To prevent permanent damage, persons adhering to a strick vegetarian diet should probably take 50 micrograms of B-12 each week while their stomach secretions are still normal."

If the symptoms of B-12 deficiency have become serious, do *not* try to treat yourself. Rush to the nearest physician for B-12 injections. He will know the amounts to give you. Leave it in his hands.

For prevention, it is better to take the entire B complex, which includes B-12, as well as the natural foods such as those mentioned above. On the label of vitamin sypplements, the vitamin may not be listed as B-12, but as cobalamin, or cynocobalamin, both synonymous. But if you are a vegetarian, do not wait for symptoms of B-12 deficiency to become apparent. As Adelle Davis writes: "Because a vegetarian diet is rich in folic acid, however, the blood remains normal and irreparable nerve damage can occur before the Vitamin B-12 deficiency is discovered."

Because folic acid can cover up or hide the adverse effects of a B-12 deficiency, only folic acid in extremely low potencies (100 micrograms) per tablet is available, if at all, at this writing, except by medical prescription.

For those who are squeamish about eating meat, fish or fowl, there are two alternatives. One is to follow the lead of the Seventh Day Adventists who have an enviable health record. They are lacto-ovo vegetarians, meaning that they use dairy products such as milk, eggs and cheese. The other alternative is to combine certain plants which, though incomplete proteins in themselves, can become complete proteins if properly combined. Complete proteins, such as meat, fish, fowl and dairy products, plus brewer's yeast, soy products, and wheat germ are already complete because they each contain *all* of the essential amino acids. But if foods which contain limited essential amino acids plus the nonessential amino acids are eaten, the body cannot synthesize protein. Strangely enough, the essential amino acids cannot be eaten piecemeal—one at one meal, another at another. *They must be eaten all at once*, or trouble can result. It usually takes a "brain" or a computer to figure out which plant foods contain which amino acids. Now help is available in a small book called *Diet for a Small Planet* (which means you), a Ballantyne paperback, written by Frances Moore Lappé for the vegetarian to show how to find enough plant protein in correct combination to supply complete proteins. However, *Vitamin B-12 is still necessary*, so eating lacto-ovo products, which are complete proteins, and which also contain Vitamin B-12, is good insurance. Brewer's yeast is also a complete protein, and some varieties are now bred to include B-12. (To identify the correct brand, read your labels at health stores.) Remember that hit-or-miss vegetarianism can have a serious delayed reaction, so it is not safe to take chances.

Vitamin/Mineral Therapy

Anemia can also result from a lack of the follöwing vitamins:
—Vitamin C
—Vitamin E
—B vitamins: thiamine (B-1), riboflavin (B-2), niacin (B-3), pyridoxine (B-6), biotin, pantothenic acid, folic acid, B-12.

Vitamins E and C can be taken separately, but it is preferable to take the entire B family (or complex). This includes all of the above B factors plus the others which are also included in liver or, if you insist upon being a vegetarian, in brewer's yeast. The only exception to this rule is folic acid, which (due to the FDA restriction) you might need separately, but cannot buy except in microscopic amounts, so you might as well get it in brewer's yeast or other forms of the entire B complex. The other exception is

B-12, which may be needed in injection form, as already discussed. Even if you are taking a single B vitamin, it is highly important to also take the entire B complex at the same time or on the same day. Too much of one factor alone, without the members of the entire B family, can cause a lopsided balance, or a shortage of another B factor, and this has led to physical disturbances.

The most recent addition to correlation of anemia and a B vitamin is a form of anemia which has been traced to a deficiency of pantothenic acid. Paul R. McGurdy, M.D., discovered that pantothenic acid therapy simultaneously cured this type of anemia and a state of deep depression.[7]

Carlton Fredericks states, "Anemia is more than a disorder; it is also an influence in aggravating associated disease, and in decreasing resistance to infection. The same B complex deficiencies which produce anemia will also interfere with phagocytosis—part of the body's defense system against bacteria."

How to Correct Simple Anemia

Safe and Unsafe Iron

If anemia is due to a lack of iron, it should be taken in *natural* organic form in food or supplements. Inorganic iron can be extremely dangerous! Adelle Davis warns in her book, *Let's Get Well,* about the dangers of ferrous sulfate and certain other iron compounds. The bad effects, she believed, may cause a destruction of protective vitamins and unsaturated fatty acids, increase a need for oxygen rather than supply it, cause serious liver damage, and during pregnancy may cause miscarriage, delayed or premature births as well as birth defects. She believed that too much ferrous sulfate is responsible for the deaths of many children annually, since 900 milligrams can be fatal. She reported that of all the iron salts, ferrous gluconate is the least toxic.

Many nutrition investigators are decrying the addition of iron to "enriched food." Bernard Bellew, M.D., writing in *Let's Live,* March, 1972, states that an overload of inorganic iron is stored in the liver, bone marrow, spleen, lungs and pancreas. He says, "There is no question that excesses of inorganic iron as used in the enrichment and fortification of foods can lead to chronic disabling and fatal disease in some people."

Beatrice Trum Hunter, writing in *Consumer Bulletin* (November, 1972) reports that bakers and millers are now hoping to quadruple the amount of iron already used in flour which ends up as bread, rolls, cookies, pastas, etc. She warns that the storage of this inorganic iron in the body can result in liver cirrhosis, diabetes, sterility and heart failure.

Food Therapy

On the other hand, *no toxicity has ever been noted from taking natural organic iron in food or supplement form.* Here are the most common foods which provide natural, organic iron. Actually, most foods, *if they are unrefined,* do contain this safe iron:

Plants

Whole grains, including wheat, whole grain cereals, brown rice and rice polishings, beets and beet greens, tomatoes, spinach (this source of iron is not well used by the body), lettuce, green leafy vegetables, cabbage, celery, parsley.

Fruit

Apples, berries, cherries, grapes, raisins, figs, dates, apricots, peaches, pears, prunes.

Meat

Beef, especially organ meats: heart, kidney. Liver, fresh, desiccated, also liquid, predigested, and unheated.

Natural iron, of course, is found in other foods, but is especially high in those named here. Liver produces more iron (also Vitamin B-12) than any known food. Next are kidney, apricots and egg yolk. Of the plants, turnip greens, a standby in the deep south, and the legumes (dried peas and beans) are rated higher than leafy greens. Blackstrap molasses is not only high in iron, but also in copper and various B vitamins as well. It is used successfully as a "tonic" for anemia. It should not be taken straight from the spoon, but can be diluted with liquid to avoid direct contact with the teeth as it otherwise can cause enamel erosion. The mouth should be rinsed immediately after taking. (Any sticky sweets, even dried fruits, will also cling to the teeth.)

Blackstrap molasses contains approximately fifteen times more iron than ordinary molasses. If you find it too bitter to take alone, or even in cooking, you can combine it with other molasses or honey. There is also a tablet made by a well-known manufacturer of natural vitamin products that has been widely used and respected for many years. This tablet contains food iron, B vitamins 1, 2, 3, 6, 12, pantothenic acid, PABA, choline, inosital and biotin; the minerals copper, magnesium, manganese and zinc. It even includes powdered edible hemoglobin, dried yeast, desiccated whole liver, natural B-12, dehydrated molasses, bone marrow and chlorophyll. In other words it contains nearly all of the elements *in natural form* known to prevent or reverse anemia. Your health store operator can help identify the brand by reading the label. (I cannot provide brand names.)

Chlorophyll is a helpful addition to this product. The late Dr. Royal Lee stated that some anemic states fail to respond to iron and B-12, but do respond when chorophyll, which sensitizes the liver, is supplied.

Beets are extremely important in anemia therapy. Beet juice contains potassium, phosphorus, calcium, sulphur, iodine, iron, copper, carbohydrates, protein, fat, Vitamins B-1, B-2, Niacin, B-6, C and Vitamin P. Dr. Sander Ferenczi of Hungary, Chief Physician of the Department of Internal Medicine, Cserna, reported that due to a high content of iron, beet juice apparently regenerates and reactivates the red blood corpuscles, supplies the body with fresh oxygen and helps the normal function of vesicular breathing. It has been known since the Middle Ages that red beet juice is associated with human blood and blood-forming properties.

Dr. Fritz Keitel, of Germany, adds, "The juice of the red beet strengthens the body's powers of resistance and has proved to be an excellent remedy for anemia, especially for children and teen-agers where other blood forming remedies have failed."

Beet juice is not always palatable. There are two varieties of lactic acid (fermented beet juice), one imported from Germany, another from Switzerland, that are not only delicious, but contain their own built-in form of acid for easy assimilation. They are available to health stores in the United States.

Minerals are another help. Kelp, and other seaweeds, are one of our richest sources of minerals. When two physicians, George L. Siefert, M.D., and H. Curtis Wood, M.D., both of Philadelphia, gave Pacific Ocean kelp (macrocystis pyrifera), three tablets daily, to 400 pregnant women, their hemoglobin rose from 65% to 83%.

In a surprising, but highly controversial, book which has only recently come to the attention of the public, though its thesis has apparently been known in Europe for many years, it is stated that the body can be its own alchemist. By taking one mineral, the body seems to be able to manufacture another mineral. For example, if you lack iron, take manganese and it can be converted to iron. The book tells the story of a pregnant woman who was found to be anemic by her doctor. Knowing that she did not like to take pills and that her metabolism was somewhat sluggish, she was told simply to take more cereals, chew them thoroughly, then make her next appointment with the doctor in the afternoon. A month later, after following these directions, the doctor found her supply of iron plentiful. The explanation is that whole grain cereals (whole wheat, brown rice, etc.) are rich in manganese which the body can convert into iron. This book, *Biological Transmutations,* is full of other exciting examples of biological transmutation, from which it gets its name. (See bibliography.)

Homeopathic Cell Salt Therapy
Another form of minerals many have found useful, and which

are easily assimilated, are the homeopathic cell salts. These come in tiny sweet pellets that one dissolves dry, on or under the tongue, without washing them down with water. They are not assimilated in the digestive tract but are absorbed directly through the tissues. Two of these cell salt minerals (there are twelve in all) are especially effective in the treatment of anemia. *Calc. Phos.* (abbreviation for Calcarea Phosphate or phosphate of lime) helps to restore a deficiency of red blood cells by nourishing the bone marrow, where blood cells are manufactured. *Ferr. Phos.* (Ferrum Phosphate, or Phosphate of Iron) helps to correct the deficiency of hemoglobin, the red coloring matter in the blood. These two cells salts have restored the blood to normal.

As an example, one homeopathic physician accepted a teen-age patient from another doctor who had been treating the 16-year-old with inorganic iron products. The girl's stomach would not tolerate or assimilate them. Consequently she was starving to death due to a lack of iron and phosphates. The homeopathic doctor prescribed for her the cell salts, *Ferr. Phos.* and *Calc. Phos.*, and she recovered within a few weeks.

Lack of the cell salt *Calc. Sulph.* is also one of the causes of anemia. In this case its deficiency contributes to a gray, pasty-appearing skin.

Nat. Phos. (Natrum Phosphate) is indicated for help in eliminating parasites.

The homeopathic cell salts are available from homeopathic pharmacies and some health stores without prescription. The dosage is listed on the label. They do not produce dangerous side effects (as compared with drugs), and are relatively inexpensive.

REFERENCES
(See *Bibliography* for fuller details.)

1. *Science Newsletter,* December 9, 1956.
2. E. Cheraskin, M.D. and W. M. Ringsdorf, Jr., D.M.D., M.S., *New Hope for Incurable Diseases.*

3. Linda Clark, *Secrets of Health and Beauty.*
4. D. C. Jarvis, M.D., *Folk Medicine.*
5. *Nutrition Reviews*, April, 1962, p. 127.
6. For herbal remedy for human parasites, look for a representative of Shaklee products in your vicinity. For herbal vermifuges for pets, write Westward Products, Box 1932, Studio City, Cal. 91604.
7. Adelle Davis, *Let's Get Well.*

5: ARTHRITIS

Arthritis can be reversed

Most practitioners believe arthritis is not a single disease, but occurs in various forms such as osteoarthritis, rheumatoid arthritis, menopausal arthritis and other forms. Even gout is considered a somewhat related disease, since for the most part, all types of arthritis affect the joints or bony structure of the body.

Jern Hamberg, M.D., of Sweden, has stated, "Arthritis is a very capricious disease. No two cases are identical. Amost every case requires an individual approach. Some cases respond very quickly, others seem to be completely incurable...or in some cases it may take a long time to bring about a cure."[1]

The orthodox medical profession has even gone so far as to say that there *is* no cure for arthritis; one must just learn to live with it. But these words of gloom need not be a final verdict. As you will see, there is real hope for sufferers from arthritis, and many people who have gone from doctor to doctor have finally, in desperation, found lasting help where they least expected it: in the field of nutrition. Those who have hopefully changed climates, tried special baths at home or at various spas, had teeth or tonsils removed because of supposed infection, or tried one drug after another including aspirin and cortisone—all with only temporary relief—should know that many sufferers have finally found permanent relief from pain, and can walk again with full use of hands, feet and back, as a result of specific, yet simple, nutritional measures. Before we look at these surprising "cures," let's look first at the cause.

Osteoarthritis

The late Dr. Royal Lee, whom many consider one of the most informed nutritionists of all time, explained that osteoarthritis is considered a "wear and tear" disease, usually associated with aging. The discomfort is felt mainly in the weight-bearing joints. Pain usually increases after exercise. Patients do not appear sick, as in the case of rheumatoid arthritis. Osteoarthritis affects the knees and elbows, as well as the lumbar and cervical areas of the spine.

Causes
According to Dr. Lee, the possible causes of osteoarthritis include:
Malnutrition
Many years of physical stress
Obesity
Alkalosis
Glandular insufficiency
Calcium deficiency
A shortage of hydrochloric acid

Symptoms (according to Dr. Lee):
Pain
Spurs (as revealed by X-rays)
Joint stiffness
Watery eyes
Dry skin and mucous membranes

Leg cramps
Bronchitis with night coughs
Wry neck
A craving for acids (due to a deficiency of hydrochloric acid)
Adrenal insufficiency
Allergies
Secondary anemia
Arteriosclerosis
Blood pressure changes
Cataracts
Gall bladder function impairment
Liver disturbance
Menopausal symptoms

Dr. Lee recommended the following treatment: natural vitamin supplements, adrenal hormones (*not* cortisone), minerals, acid in some form to help the assimilation of calcium, plus fresh raw fruits, green leafy vegetables, and whole grain foods.

Rheumatoid Arthritis

Dr. Lee explained that 80% of rheumatoid arthritis cases occur in women, usually before the age of forty. It apparently affects joints of fingers, wrists, knees and feet. This form of arthritis is called the "cooked food disease."

Causes (according to Dr. Lee)
May be of allergic origin
Hormonal imbalance—(adrenal, liver, pituitary and sex glands)
Lack of raw foods

Symptoms
Anemia
Colitis
Constipation
Pain, especially in back ligaments

Gout
Gall bladder disturbance
Low blood pressure
Deformed hands and feet
Edema in ankles
Neurasthenic symptoms, with attacks often preceded by emotional stress
Absence of hydrochloric
acid

Treatment

Dr. Lee recommended the use of raw, fresh fruits and vegetables, including potato and raw potato juice. He recommended protein: fresh fish and fowl, plus brown rice and a *low intake of carbohydrates*. Also natural, fresh fruits, plus acid in some form.

Dr. Lee considered yogurt helpful, due to the acid as well as calcium content, especially in cases of constipation. However, he warned against citrus fruits (except lemon in small amounts) and refined sugar (even dried natural dates, figs, and honey), or refined carbohydrates, all of which he found will increase pain.

Dr. Paavo O. Airola agrees with Dr. Lee. He states, "An unbalanced diet of devitalized, overprocessed, overcooked and overrefined denatured foods . . . together with other negative environmental factors, brings about a general deterioration of health, biochemical inbalances, and systemic disturbances . . . (which) eventually lead to . . . pathological changes in the joints and tissues of the body." Dr. Airola points an accusing finger especially to foodless items including sugar, soft drinks, sweets, pastries, pies, etc.[1]

Although in advanced cases of arthritis, where physical disfigurement of joints takes place, the greatest burden for the afflicted to bear is pain. No wonder an arthritic will seek a panacea, a drug, *anything* that will promise relief from the agonizing pain. Some people have taken cortisone only to find that a moon face, excessive growth of facial hair in women, edema, diabetes, high blood pressure, peptic ulcers, spinal calcification, mental disturbances and psychoses or nerve degeneration can and do result as serious side effects of this drug.

Many people, frantic to be relieved from pain, gobble down aspirin. Aspirin does relieve pain, but masks the symptoms, and can eventually cause internal bleeding, edema, heart disturbances, even incoherence and confusion. In fact, aspirin can cause poisoning so severe as to bring about serious changes in kidneys, liver and brain.[2]

There are better ways to cope with this disease.

Calcium is a Must

According to Carlton Fredericks, Ph.D., and Adelle Davis, there is a great need in arthritics for calcium and calcium foods, despite the fact that many orthodox doctors warn their patients not to take them, believing that the calcium will merely pile up in the joints. This appears to be an erroneous conclusion. Dr. Fredericks says that if you do not take calcium, the system will steal it from bones in other parts of the body in order to protect against convulsions, which can occur if the calcium in the blood becomes too low. Then, by weakening the bones, the calcium shortage can lead to osteoporosis as well as osteoarthritis. Dr. Fredericks says you should not stop calcium, but take more!

Many people are puzzled because they believe that taking calcium will cause it to be deposited in their joints. If this occurs, however, it is due to another cause. *Acid is needed to dissolve calcium* so that it will *not* turn into deposits. If you do not believe this, drop a bone meal tablet in a glass of water or milk and watch what happens. Nothing. It will probably still be intact several days later. But if you add some apple cider vinegar, or hydrochloric acid (a natural digestant manufactured by the body but lacking in some people), or add a high potency Vitamin C tablet, the calcium will begin breaking down. The process is the same in the body. If the calcium is dissolved within the body, as it should be, the chances are that it will be held in solution and distributed where it is needed—to glands, tissues and blood, and *not* pile up in the joints where it is not wanted.

This was the thesis of the late D. C. Jarvis, M.D., who used apple cider vinegar in feed and water for cattle, and later for people, to prevent, or reverse, calcium deposits. To demonstrate, he put some vinegar and water in a tea kettle, the inside surface of which had become encrusted with calcium and other mineral deposits. Left for a number of hours, the vinegar water dissolved all of the deposits. The process, he pointed out, is applicable to the body.[3] He wrote:

Vermont folk medicine does not recognize a difference among bursitis, rheumatoid arthritis, osteoarthritis and muscular rheumatism ... they are all treated the same way.

Vermont folk medicine believes that the treatment of arthritis begins in the stomach ... when the acid (hydrochloric) is diminished in quantity or is absent, as it may be, there is no check on the growth of microorganisms in the stomach.... People with arthritis are usually classified as calcium-deficient, even though they tend to accumulate calcium deposits. Vermont folk medicine says they are not making hydrochloric acid in the stomach, or else the amount made is too small ... normal calcium metabolism is so highly dependent upon this acid that when there is a lack of it a disturbed calcium metabolism is inevitable.

In treating arthritis, folk medicine first prescribes two teaspoons of apple cider vinegar and two of honey in a glass of water with each meal, sipped like coffee.

Autopsies of cows revealed that vinegar previously added to the ration had removed the calcium deposits in blood vessel walls.[4]

Robert Bingham, M.D. reports in the *Journal of Applied Nutrition,* Winter, 1972 issue, that many hundreds of patients have testified to relief from their arthritic symptoms by this method of using vinegar.

Dr. E. Hugh Tuckey had successful results with arthritics, actually getting them back to work by giving them acid in the form of hydrochloric acid. (For Dr. Tuckey's method, dosage and types of HCL to use, see my book, *Secrets of Health and Beauty.*[5]

Adelle Davis, in order to supply acid for arthritics, recommended massive doses of Vitamin C (ascorbic acid) coupled with a calcium tablet with each dose.[6]

Other minerals besides calcium are considered necessary for arthritis. In fact there is conjecture that arthritis may be a general mineral-deficiency disease. Dr. Bernard Spur, a Danish biochemist, believes that a deficiency of minerals is involved in all rheumatic diseases. . . . Dr. Jarvis recommended kelp tablets. You also may have read the story of George W. Crane, M.D.'s 96-year-old father-in-law, who was a wheelchair victim of arthritis before his recovery, which was due to adding sea water (a source of all minerals) to his daily drinking water.[7]

Another source of minerals is the Schuessler homeopathic cell salts. If you cannot find the all-in-one product (there are twelve individual cell salts) at a homeopathic pharmacy or health store in your area, write for information to the Standard Homeopathic Pharmacy, P.O. Box 61067, Los Angeles, Ca. 90061.

Vitamins

One nutritional clinic treats osteoarthritis with high calcium (bonemeal or liquid calcium—ask your health store), high protein, high vitamin intake, including *all* vitamins—A, E, B complex and others—as well as unsaturated fats. The clinic's success in patient improvement is excellent.

In rheumatoid arthritis the adrenal glands are involved. Unfortunately the usual orthodox approach is the use of cortisone, but as already mentioned, the side effects can be devastating. There is a safer remedy, namely, the B vitamin, pantothenic acid, which affects the adrenal glands favorably. If a person is also plagued with multiple allergies, it is a sign that his adrenals are malfunctioning. So pantothenic acid can come to the rescue for both allergies and this type of arthritis.

The adrenals are a storage depot for Vitamin C. In case of prolonged tension, or even in minor or temporary stress, such as a quarrel with your husband or wife, or in the case of sudden shock, the adrenals are deprived of their store of Vitamin C almost within seconds. I have written elsewhere about the man whose wife ran away with another man. The next day he was in a wheelchair, an arthritis victim. Since disturbances of the adrenals have also been found to affect loss of hair color in animals, it may explain why some people, after sudden and severe shock, have turned white-haired overnight.

Dr. E. C. Barton-Wright, a microbiologist, believes that arthritis is neither a bacterial infection nor an auto-immune disease. He is convinced that it is a vitamin-deficiency disease which can be prevented or relieved by a diet containing adequate quantities of pantothenic acid. Dr. W. A. Eliot and Dr. Barton-Wright, both of England, were the first to show that the pantothenic acid content of the blood of persons suffering from rheumatoid arthritis was lower than that in healthy individuals. (*Here's Health*, Feb. 1975.)

Three other London researchers also found that arthritis imbalance could be helped by pantothenic acid plus royal jelly and cystine (an amino acid present in brewer's yeast). Twice daily they gave arthritic patients 25 mg. of calcium pantothenate and 15 mg. of cystine. There was no improvement for four to eight weeks. Just as the patient was deciding the treatment was useless, symptoms disappeared overnight. The doctors believed that this routine, reduced to one tablet of pantothenic acid twice daily, must be maintained indefinitely to prevent return of symptoms.[8] Any single B vitamin should be accompanied by the entire B complex from brewer's yeast, liver, or both, to avoid imbalance of the other Vitamin B factors.

Some investigators have called attention to the fact that arthritis is a resentment disease. The arthritic, suffering from malfunctioning adrenals, may appear faultfinding, critical of others and of everything, and often does a continuous slow burn of resentment. Whether the negative emotional state of mind, or the arthritis, occurs first is not clear, but the problem is noticeable in many sufferers.

In addition to pantothenic acid to help repair the adrenal

glands, the entire Vitamin C complex in *large* amounts is advocated by nutritionists, especially for rheumatoid arthritis. (Small amounts may worsen the condition, according to Carlton Fredericks.) The deficiency of the C complex (bioflavonoids) is also a factor in eye hemorrhaging which may occur in some arthritics but responds dramatically within days to high doses of bioflavonoids. Dr. Fredericks' suggestions for rheumatoid arthritis include a hypoglycemic (low carbohydrate) diet, since a high carbohydrate diet aggravates rheumatoid arthritis. He also suggests the use of vegetable oils such as wheat germ oil (others recommend cod liver oil), Vitamins E, C, bioflavonoids, pantothenic acid and eggs—at least two daily. On this diet, Dr. Fredericks cites the case of a man, an arthritic victim, who was able to abandon his wheelchair.

John M. Ellis, M.D., author of a book explaining his great success with the use of Vitamin B-6, finds that approximately 50 mg. of B-6 daily specifically helps arthritis "spurs" and finger stiffness.[9] He also recommends eating pecans daily.

Joe D. Nichols, M.D., head of Natural Food Associates, in his book[10] cites the case of one of his patients whose fingers had become so stiff he could no longer hold a golf club. When Dr. Nichols put him on a complete diet of natural, organic food, much of it raw, Vitamin B-6 (plus a supply of all of the B vitamins), the man was back on the golf course within three weeks. His hand stiffness had disappeared.

Herbs

Some herbs have been found helpful in arthritis. Ash, lucerne and comfrey have been mentioned in one herb book.[11] Richard Lucas[12] mentions celery, also sassafras, which is well known as a cleanser.

The Orientals occasionally use Ginseng with good effects for arthritis.

All of these herbs have usually been taken in the form of tea. But a new, exciting and surprising use of herbs for arthritis, as well as for many other complaints, has recently come to light.

Maurice Mességué, author of a No. 1 bestselling book in France, now published in this country,[13] had had dramatic cures by using herbs in a different way. M. Mességué, who has treated thousands of patients suffering from many ailments with a combination of herbs, each chosen for the specific condition, uses them not internally, but externally in hand and foot baths, as hot as can be tolerated, for only 8 minutes each. Whatever their ailments, people ranging from kings to paupers have reported excellent results from this therapy. For arthritis, M. Mességué names six herbs: Garlic (1 whole head, crushed), Greater Celandine leaves (one handful), Nettle (whole plant, two handfuls), Dandelion (whole plant, one handful), Meadowsweet (flowers, one handful), Buttercup (whole plant, one handful), most of them easily obtained from the garden or herb companies. He explains in the book how to prepare the infusion for the 8-minute hand and foot baths. The book, an autobiography, is fascinating to read.

Another herb has proven helpful. One woman wrote me that she had suffered from pain and disability for years as a result of advanced osteoarthritis. The inflammation was in her neck, jaw and back and was spreading to her hip, as established by X-rays. The doctors were unable to help her, she says. Then she discovered nutrition and natural remedies. She writes, "Finally the Indian herbal remedy, Chaparral (also known as *gobernadora* or creosote bush) worked like a miracle. The pain was soothingly and gently relieved—within one week to ten days." She took two tablets a day, she wrote, one at breakfast, the other with dinner.

Prior to taking the Chaparral, this woman, 58 years old, said that the pain and inflammation were so bad she had difficulty dressing, reaching for things, and walking. The pain was even too severe in a seated position for sewing and reading. She also felt exhausted all of the time."After using the tablets, I tried the tea form," she wrote, "but found it ineffective. Then I returned to the tablets: 7½ gr., with 2 tablets at each meal and at bedtime. Recently, it stopped working. The pain came back. I stopped taking it, waited a week, and resumed it again, and again it is working. I am also taking B complex, calcium, Vitamin D, kelp, magnesium and various herb teas. I had taken the other teas before trying Chaparral, and they did not help me. But the Chaparral itself did the job!" (This herb can be found in most health stores.)

Mike Spencer, former editor of *Let's Live* Magazine, reports in the February, 1975 issue of the use of a recent discovery: yucca. Tests show that about 20 percent of arthritics tested had a complete remission of joint pains, minimal swelling and inflammation. About 30 percent showed improvement and relief of some joint pains, stiffness and swelling. The remaining 50 percent detected no changes, but in this group some had tried it for only two weeks.

Yucca tablets are now available from health stores who can order them from Botanical Products, Inc., 17656 Avenue 168, Porterville, California 93257.

More Hope for Arthritics

There are some investigators who believe that arthritis is not only a "cooked and refined food disease," but a disease of toxicity. Remembering that pain is the greatest burden of all, the stiffness next, it is encouraging to learn that two doctors have found a way not only to relieve, but to *remove* pain quickly and naturally, without drugs. Paavo O. Airola, N.D. reports in his book[1] "cures" for arthritis which are taking place in Europe daily at various spas dedicated to this type of healing. Both the Bircher-Benner Clinic in Zurich, Switzerland, and the famed Buchinger Clinic in Bad Pyrmont, Germany, under the aegis of Dr. Otto Buchinger Jr., M.D., perhaps the world's outstanding expert on fasting, are attracting patients and nutritionists alike. There are other spas and sanitaria which are having similar results. The pattern that links these spas or sanitaria is the use of certain carefully planned fasts (this does not mean just water, but juices, herb teas, etc.) which are given *under medical supervision*.

Dr. Airola, mentioned above, says that raw diets, or special types of fasting (or both) can eliminate the waste and sluggishness in the body by a cleansing, detoxifying and purifying process. When this cleansing is sufficient, he says, pain stops, a person can give up his crutches, and in some people this may happen within days or a few weeks. If the person continues to live on the correct diet the trouble may never return. Dr. Airola gives many case histories of such people in his book.

Not all types of fasts are safe. Fasting with water only, *without the supervision of a doctor* is especially dangerous because the poisons in the body are released so quickly and suddenly that the person may poison himself. Cases of death have occurred as a result. Fasts using fruit juices and raw foods are safer, but these fasts, too, should also be supervised, or at least be clearly outlined by experts who have used them successfully for therapeutic purposes in thousands of cases.

In his book, Dr. Airola tells of some actual cases of arthritis cures in which the patients who had suffered for years, were pain-ridden and unable to walk. These patients, within a few weeks, became pain-free, were no longer stiff and returned home in good health that continued as long as the diet, largely of raw foods, was followed.

You need not take the next plane for Europe if you cannot afford it. Dr. Airola's book tells you the exact method and diet used at the European spas which you can use in your own home.

Most exciting of all, in my opinion, is a recent book by Giraud W. Campbell, D.O.[14] that tells of amazing arthritis cures in *seven days*! One example is that of a 42-year-old housewife who had been arthritic for six years, and bedridden for six months. Without any drugs, including aspirin (which Dr. Campbell usually tapers off in his patients, though it was not necessary in this case), the pain was all gone in seven days. In two weeks the woman was out of bed, walking, and had regained the use of her formerly useless hands.

Dr. Campbell makes little distinction between osteoarthritis and rheumatoid arthritis, since his seven-day program is prescribed for both types. His program is, briefly, one day only of fasting, followed by a total natural *raw food diet* with no refined, preserved or cooked foods at all. (He points an accusing finger to the additives in our processed foods.) Later, vitamins and minerals are added. That is it! But you will need to read his book to learn exactly how to use his program.

For those who may scoff, there is another dramatic surprise in the book. You may say, "O.K. This program relieves you of pain, but what about deformities? Won't they be always with us?"

Dr. Campbell says, "The cause of the weakening of the bones and joints is due to wrong diet." Thus he not only believes, but has proof that the *right* diet can repair the damage in the bones and joints. He shows before-and-after X-rays of hip joints, knee joints and spinal deterioration revealing repair of the arthritic damage that occurred within six to eight months! Believe me, anyone who is a suffering arthritic is shortchanging himself if he does not read—and follow—the valuable information in this book. There are cases galore of those who had gone from doctor to doctor and hospital to hospital with no results, but who, as a desperate last resort, followed Dr. Campbell's method and not only became well, but stayed well. This should end this poppycock, once and for all, that nutrition is useless, as well as the myth that "there is no cure for arthritis." Read about it and try it for yourself instead of giving in to pain and discouragement.

A new book, *Overcoming Arthritis*,[15] by Max Warmbrand, D.O., N.D., D.C., cites many cases of cures following a detoxification program and a diet of raw foods, plus exercises.

Sometimes, although the *whole* program previously outlined is necessary to bring arthritis under control, if the person has been on a reasonably good diet as well as stress-free, a shortcut can bring results. For example, I have told elsewhere of a friend who was a piano teacher. During the summer she developed great pain and stiffness in her fingers, making it almost impossible to demonstrate correct piano playing to her pupils. When she learned that citrus fruit can increase arthritic symptoms and pain, she realized that during the hot weather she drank large amounts of grapefruit juice. When she ceased using the grapefruit juice, her hands returned to normal.

Another example is too good not to share with you. Ruth

Stout, sister of the late Rex Stout, the "whodunit writer," and an author in her own right, discovered a method of composting her organic garden which made gardening almost work-free. As a result, she has written several charming books: *How to Have a Green Thumb Without an Aching Back, Gardening Without Work,* and others (available through book stores). I know for a fact that, now in her early nineties, she has embraced a good nutritional diet for many years. But recently I received a letter from her that contained some surprising arthritis information.

She told me she had read (but does not recall where) about a diet that cured arthritis. She wrote, "This diet cured me almost immediately—in less than two weeks, with no pain at all afterwards. I kept quiet about it for a while because I thought everyone would say I couldn't have had arthritis, although two doctors said it was.

"Then, eight months ago my milkman got arthritis so badly the doctor said he would have to give up his job driving the truck. I told him about the diet, and in ten days he was back on his feet and still is. Yesterday a newspaper reporter came to my house to talk about arthritis and my milkman showed up. The reporter took a picture of both of us sitting on the couch looking happily well.

"I also have told about this diet on the radio and have received many good reports from others. The diet is very simple: just eat pecans, brewer's yeast, wheat germ, bananas and avocado, plus anything else you want. Each day we ate 12 pecan halves, one banana, a heaping teaspoon each of wheat germ and brewer's yeast. We ate almost no avocado because we couldn't get them in the Northeast. At the beginning, we both had awful pains in our back and legs. After we began the diet, the pain left within two weeks. Pain has never come back, although my trouble started three years ago, and the milkman's a year ago."

The only explanation I can provide for this simple diet is that both pecans and bananas are rich in Vitamin B-6. Wheat germ is rich in Vitamin E, and avocado contains unsaturated fatty acids. And all the others—B vitamins, protein (amino acids) and minerals—are in brewer's yeast. I am sure Ruth took Vitamin C on her own, and knowing her, she also probably converted the milkman to a good nutritional diet.

Whatever the explanation, recalling the statement by Dr. Hamberg at the beginning of this chapter that arthritis is a capricious disease, Ruth Stout is proof that it can be licked. It couldn't happen to a grander gal, who is in her nineties and still going strong!

I received a letter from a woman who has tried this diet. She wrote me: "When I read about Ruth Stout's diet, I immediately started the banana, pecan, wheat germ and brewer's yeast. I have had arthritis since I was eleven years old (at which time I had rheumatic fever). I am now sixty-two.

"Here's the good news: after four weeks on the diet, I have not had an ache or a pain from arthritis since. It is like a miracle because prior to going on that fabulous diet, I had pain practically every day for forty-nine years too long. I have told *so* many people what I did because I want everyone to feel as well as I do.

"I also added further instructions mentioned elsewhere and use the fiber-free alfalfa concentrate made from the seeds. I am continuing this in order to maintain my 'no ache' status."

A final shortcut is the use of the 100% fiber-free alfalfa concentrate tablet mentioned above. This type of alfalfa tablet contains all the oil soluble vitamins, plus protein and chlorophyll, a potent detoxifier. Not only has sludged blood responded to this treatment, but as the toxicity leaves the body, so does the pain. It has been tested and enthusiastically acclaimed by approximately 5,000 people. Results, when taken in sufficient dosage, have occurred in a short time, ranging from a few days to a month, depending upon the toxic condition of the individual.[16]

One case which I know of personally is that of a 36-year-old man. His swollen knees and excruciating pain had kept him out of work for six months, threatening his income for himself, his wife and child. After trying "everything" he had heard of in the field of natural therapy, he finally went to two orthodox physicians, considered experts on arthritis. They diagnosed his condition as acute rheumatoid arthritis, prescribed drugs, and hot baths for pain relief. He sat day after day with his lower legs submerged in the hottest possible water, while tears due to the pain streamed down his face.

Then someone told him about the alfalfa tablets. Since he had already had so many disappointments, he did not expect any relief. However, a therapist who had watched results in many others told him that the tablets, in double the daily dosage mentioned on the label, should bring relief within a week. This did not happen; it took one and one-half weeks! By that time the man's pain and swelling were gone and he was back to work. Since then, he and his wife have told hundreds of sufferers about the alfalfa treatment, with good results. There is no hocus-pocus about this treatment. It is just another of nature's plants which nourishes and detoxifies simultaneously.

REFERENCES
(See *Bibliography* for fuller details.)

1. Paavo O. Airola, N.D., *There Is a Cure for Arthritis*.
2. *Journal of the American Medical Association*, November 15, 1947.
3. D. C. Jarvis, M.D., *Folk Medicine*.
4. D. C. Jarvis, M.D., *Arthritis and Folk Medicine*.
5. Linda Clark, *Secrets of Health and Beauty*.
6. Adelle Davis, *Let's Eat Right to Keep Fit*.
7. Linda Clark, *Know Your Nutrition*.
8. *Medical World News*, October 7, 1966.
9. John M. Ellis, M.D., *The Doctor Who Looked at Hands*.
10. Joe D. Nichols, M.D., *Please, Doctor, Do Something!*
11. Joseph Kadans, N.D., Ph.D., *Encyclopedia of Medicinal Herbs*.
12. Richard Lucas, *Common and Uncommon Uses of Herbs for Healthful Living*.
13. Maurice Mességué, *Of Men and Plants: The Autobiography of the World's Most Famous Plant Healer*.
14. Giraud W. Campbell, D.O., with Robert Stone, *A Doctor's Proven Cure for Arthritis*.

15. Max Warmbrand, N.D., D.O., D.C., *Overcoming Arthritis*.
16. For further information about alfalfa, write: Frank Lachle, 117 E. Lake St., Watsonville, Cal. 95076.

6: ASTHMA — EMPHYSEMA

Respiratory diseases, especially asthma, chronic bronchitis, bronchial asthma and emphysema, are increasing by leaps and bounds all over the world. The common denominator underlying these disturbances seems to be air pollution, which may not necessarily *cause* the conditions but apparently aggravates them in susceptible people. Smoking does not help.

These conclusions have been reached by Dr. Murray Spotnitz, of Fitzsimons General Hospital, Denver, who found that air pollution may intensify the lung problems if already present.[1] However, dogs exposed to a high concentration of sulphur dioxide, one of the components of polluted air, were found to develop abnormalities in lung function, according to Dr. Richard Martin, of McGill University, Montreal.[2] Lung disturbances have also been traced to car exhaust pollutants: hydrocarbons, carbon monoxide, as well as nitrous oxide, all found in polluted air. Even nonsmoker's can breathe in pollutants which are the equivalent of smoking twenty cigarettes a day.[3]

There are some helpful remedies which can be used for these lung ailments, but in order to derive the greatest and quickest help from them, you will need to understand what happens within your body when you contract asthma, emphysema, or related disturbances. "To be forewarned is to be forearmed." Let's look at asthma first.

Asthma

In asthma, victims appear to be gasping for air. Actually, according to asthma specialists, asthmatics have more trouble *exhaling* than *inhaling* because the air passages of the small bronchii become clogged and constricted with mucus, narrowing the passages, thus making it hard for the person to exhale.[4]

Asthma has long been considered to be initiated by psychological or emotional reactions, or allergies. But other factors have been observed, too. A falling barometer has been noted prior to some asthmatic attacks, and certain geographical climates or locations were credited with relief for asthmatics until pollution became a world-wide problem: no area may now be permanently immune.[5]

Another unsuspected antagonist in some cases of already existing asthma is acetylsalicylic acid, better known as aspirin. Even drugs containing aspirin should be watched for. Physicians may be unaware that some drugs contain aspirin, and patients should read labels of over-the-counter drugs to see if aspirin (often listed as acetylsalicylic acid) is present. The warning comes from Dr. Constantine J. Falliers, director of a private asthma and allergy clinic in Denver. Dr. Falliers has made a study of 1,298 children over a period of fourteen years, and though not all of the asthmatics were found susceptible to aspirin, those who were, developed common allergic or adverse reactions including hives, swollen lips and eyes, bronchial spasms, wheezing, and lowered blood pressure.[6]

Still more surprising is the discovery that intestinal parasites have been found to produce asthma symptoms such as wheezing, coughing and shortness of breath.[7]

A strange new cause of asthma, now called meat wrapper's asthma, was discovered by three California doctors. The patients developed severe respiratory problems following the cutting of polyvinyl plastic film with a hot wire. The workers had been employed as wrappers for six to ten years without respiratory disturbance until they began using the plastic. There were no special means of ventilation provided to remove fumes. (*Journal of the American Medical Association*, November 5, 1973.)

The late Dr. Royal Lee, nutrition expert, pointed an accusing finger at malnutrition in general, with adrenal insufficiency, hypoglycemia, and intolerances for carbohydrates as specific factors leading to asthma in adults. He found that the older the patient, the more intractible the asthma. He also believed that in young children, the major cause of asthma was due to allergy. But there is a more recent discovery, little known, which shows that there is an operating factor in people themselves, which predisposes many individuals, adults and children, to asthma, and that this factor, properly recognized and treated, can reverse many cases, whether the cause be emotional or physical.

Asthma may have been too long considered an incurable disease because it has resisted such usual treatments as antibiotics, antihistamines, and psychotherapy (which may supply relief, but not cure). Now comes a new breakthrough with a nutritional treatment by a physician who has used it successfully for bronchial asthma, chronic rhinitis, chronic dermatitis and hay fever.

Carl J. Reich, M.D., of Canada, considers asthma a maladaptive state of the body, due to deficiency of certain nutritional elements. He feels that though stress may indeed be a large factor in asthma, the chronic deficiency of certain nutritional elements underlies the basic problem which is triggered by stress. Because of this deficiency, Dr. Reich believes that the body cannot defend itself and muscle spasms and constriction in the lungs result. He not only believes this, he has *proved* it.

Dr. Reich has used Vitamin A, Vitamin D and bone meal in treating some 5,000 cases, with success in 75% of adult cases and 90% success with children ranging from age one to ten. Dr.

Reich finds that Vitamin A helps to keep the mucous membranes moist, rather than becoming hard and scaly, and people may vary in their need of Vitamin A. Those who smoke or live in highly polluted areas seem to need more Vitamin A than others. Dr. Reich begins his treatment with high dosages of Vitamins A and D, usually in the form of natural fish liver oil (which contains both vitamins) as well as generous amounts of bone meal to provide mineral content. He tapers off the high dosages as the disturbances are brought under control.

He has tested his results not only in unrelated individuals, but in entire families.

In one family, five members, ranging through ages 59, 34, 22, 9, and 6, were suffering from chronic asthma, rhinitis and other related diseases. Dr. Reich found all deficient in Vitamins A and D, as well as in minerals. After this nutritional treatment was begun, improvement was noted within as short a time as three days, followed by continued gradual improvement. Relief occurred in leg aches, overweight, indigestion, headaches, dizziness and skin disturbances, as well as in asthma symptoms.

In another family, a six-year-old boy had been a chronic asthmatic since age two. He suffered from repetitive colds, wheezing and asthmatic spells lasting from seven to ten days. In thirty-one days of Dr. Reich's treatments, the boy no longer wheezed on exertion and could play outdoors for an entire day without developing an asthma attack. Within seven months, he had had only one cold and one asthma spell. Two other children in the same family, also chronic asthmatics, responded favorably to the nutritional treatments. The father, thirty-one years old, and an asthmatic, was so impressed with the results on his children that he asked Dr. Reich for help, too.

In still another family four members were asthmatic. The father, age twenty-four, had had asthma for two years. After several weeks of nutritional treatment, he had fewer spells, more energy and more "wind." Approximately a month later, he was considered close to being 100% cured and was able to chase his horses into the barn without wheezing, formerly an impossible task. The asthmatic twelve-year-old son was able to take part in karate and football after only two months of treatment. An eight-year-old in the same family with a history of asthma since age two, progressed to the point where night wheezing, coughs and nervousness also disappeared in two months of treatment.[8]

Dr. Reich concludes, "Only about 25% of the distress currently experienced in the so-called 'allergic diseases' is due to true allergic reaction, whereas 75% is due to nutritional deficiency reaction."[9]

Remedies for breathing problems and elimination of excess mucus will be discussed later. Now let's look at emphysema.

Emphysema

Emphysema is becoming epidemic. Most people and many doctors do not know what to do about it. One physicians told me, "I advise a good diet, plenty of rest, and don't worry too much about it."

But another physician disagreed. He said, "When a patient comes to my office panting for breath after walking only ten steps, I know it is too late. Emphysema, if not caught early, can be a killer."

Cases of death from emphysema are mounting alarmingly throughout the world. The increase of emphysema (as well as bronchitis and other respiratory diseases) has been traced to smog, as previously supposed, but also *directly to nuclear fall-out.* This is not guesswork, but the result of tests reported by Dr. Ernest J. Sternglass, professor of radiation physics, University of Pittsburgh. After extensive tests of both smog and fall-out, he stated, "All evidence pointed to radioactive air pollution, both from fall-out and nuclear power plants, as the greatest single contributor to the rise of chronic lung disease around the world."[10,11] Other researchers believe that emphysema is accelerated by cigarette smoke and other irritants. A 1971 study of 50,000 emphysema patients showed that men between the ages of forty and fifty-nine, who smoked a pack or more of cigarettes a day, were sixteen times more likely to have emphysema than those who did not smoke regularly.[12]

Emphysema differs from asthma in several respects. One difference is that in the former, small balloon-like sacs in the lungs, known as the alveoli, can no longer expel air and mucus collects because of loss of elasticity. Air can get into the lungs and alveoli rather easily when normal. These alveoli resemble a bunch of grapes. But as emphysema (which means "inflation") progresses, the sacs blow up larger, lose their elasticity, become over-stretched and begin to resemble small balloons which can no longer empty easily. An emphysema victim finds it more and more difficult to exhale; the advanced emphysema victim pants for air upon the slightest exertion.

Theodore Berland and Gordon L. Snider, M.D., say, "The cough of emphysema is not the juicy cough of asthma or bronchitis, in which sputum is spit up, but a dry, nonproductive cough. But, as in bronchitis and asthma, the small airways of the lungs—irritated by cigarette smoke and air pollutants—become inflamed and offer tremendous resistance to exhaled air. This is complicated further by the thick mucus collecting in the airways, due to absence of cilia (small hairlike projections present in normal conditions) to move it upward."[13]

An expert in lung diseases is qualified to diagnose your condition correctly by eliciting information as well as by taking certain tests. Diagnosis of emphysema is not a reliable do-it-yourself project, nor are symptoms something to be shrugged off. When such breathing symptoms strike, *immediate* action is called for. However, once you are aware of the correct diagnosis, there are remedies you can use at home. By catching it in time, the outlook can be hopeful.

Remedies for Asthma and Emphysema

Look for possible causes of antagonists in cases of asthma and eliminate them if possible. Since smoking irritates the bronchii, and may encourage an asthma attack, it merely makes sense to give it up. It may be well worth trading smoking for better health or even life itself. If an allergy may cause an attack, search for the offender and either avoid it or learn how to develop an immunity to it. (See "Allergies" in an earlier chapter.)

Watch out for drugs! Some drugs merely mask symptoms but do not really improve your condition. Epinephrine is often given to relax spasms and is also found in devices called inhalers. Serious side effects have been credited to drug inhalers. Actually, epinephrine is a natural body hormone secreted by the adrenal glands. Pantothenic acid (a B vitamin) or Vitamin C can be safer as well as acting as a natural antihistamine. (Described under nutritional remedies.)

Tension and stress can also cause the smooth muscles of the bronchii to develop spasms.

The *Well Body Book* states that the body can and will actually stop the asthmatic attack by itself. "The changes which cause the narrowing of the air passages are reversible. Your body can widen these tubes just as it can narrow them, by relaxing the smooth muscles in the bronchii, reabsorbing the body fluids and coughing up the mucus . . . many people have cured themselves of asthma, by preventing colds, avoiding fatigue, getting adequate sleep, or doing relaxation exercises and consciously letting go of the tense areas, as well as of each part of the body."[4]

Nutritional Remedies

Tests in the U.S. and Japan show that protective barriers can be developed by increasing body resistance through improved nutrition and supplements.[3] Vitamin E is one such factor which helps to improve the distribution of oxygen to various parts of the body. Various studies have shown the effects of Vitamin E on animals:

Vitamin E (and C) help inhibit damage to lung membranes after exposure to nitrogen dioxide (found in smog).

Effect of these smog pollutants may be partially prevented by prior treatments with large doses of Vitamin E.

Rats deficient in Vitamin E were more susceptible to ozone than Vitamin E-supplemented rats.[13]

M.I.T. scientists found that the combination of Vitamins A and E has protected lungs against air pollution. Those animals noticeably deficient in Vitamin A exhibited hard, scaly, thick lung cells, which improved within eighteen hours after the administration of Vitamin A. As for Vitamin E, studies in three centers found that rats given extra Vitamin E when they were exposed to smog, lived twice as long as those without it.[14]

Since cadmium and radioactive fall-out have been found to cause emphysema, there is a nutritional remedy for both, as discovered by McGill University, Montreal, Canada. This remedy, which prevents or neutralizes these dangerous substances in the body, as tested by McGill, is a form of kelp, known as alginate. Health food stores carry this product in different forms: magnesium alginate, sodium alginate, etc. The word "alginate" is the clue that the base is from kelp, which is the substance found to do the job. Alginates are available at health stores.

Ascorbic acid has prevented attacks, if taken in regular doses ranging from 500 to 1500 mg., or stopped attacks by injection of 200 to 300 mg. every fifteen minutes.[15]

Irwin Stone also reports the good effects of Vitamin C for asthmatics. Mr. Stone writes, "Asthmatics have a greater requirement for ascorbic acid." It seems to be useful in preventing constriction and spasms of the smooth muscles, as established by studies with guinea pigs. Ascorbic acid can play a dual role; as an antihistamine, if the asthmatic attack is due to an allergy (as it often is), or to relax the smooth muscle walls of the small bronchii, during as attack which interferes with breathing.[16]

As for emphysema, Dr. Lee believed that an overalkaline state in the body aggravates the condition. Smog has been found to cause overalkalinity as well as lung abnormalities and other ailments.

One woman wrote me that she and her husband living in Southern California both suffered from nausea in the late afternoon on smoggy days. She also developed knee pains. Some people might well consider the following harmless remedy for smog poisoning.

A horse, whose hair was falling rapidly, was diagnosed as having smog poisoning. To correct overalkalinity, also present, apple cider vinegar was added to the horse's drinking water. Hair falling stopped, grew in again, and the horse recovered. This supplies a tip to people: Add a little apple cider vinegar (enough to taste pleasant) to your drinking water and sip it with each meal. Adding a bit of honey can also help the body to immunize itself against bacteria, according to Russian research.

Remedies for Mucus

To help combat mucus, drinking fenugreek tea or taking fenugreek tablets have been found helpful. Like most other remedies, this does not produce overnight results. It may have to be continued for several weeks.

Remember that mucus, per se, is not something to be feared. The body manufactures it to protect mucous membranes from various irritants. It is only when excess mucus develops that its removal is necessary. This is sometimes called catarrh. It can clog up sinuses, or as in bronchial catarrh, clog up lung areas.

Vitamin C, in large doses, has dispersed mucus, according to Fred R. Klenner, M.D., who used it as a remedy in one child suffering from nasal diphtheria. Three children were afflicted with this disease simultaneously. The one who received high dosages of Vitamin C, recovered. The other two who went to other doctors not prescribing Vitamin C, died. Diphtheria has long been considered an "old time" disease, but it seems to be making a reappearance. The usual form in which a "false membrane" appears in the throat, has responded to lemon juice, taken straight, after medical help believed there was no hope for recovery. The patient got well.[17] Lemon juice, of course, is high in Vitamin C.

A Japanese study has revealed that taking 100 I.U. of Vitamin E daily for from five to seven days decreased allergy symptoms from 33% to 37% of the patients treated.[18]

Watch out for drugs! Drug antihistamines can have dangerous side effects: while driving cars, or when given in the form of nosedrops. Although they do dry up mucus, they also plug the bronchii.[19]

A baby, eight months old, given a common drug, *tetrahydrozoline*, for nasal congestion, lost consciousness, was rushed to a hospital, where it took three to four hours of continuous oxygen administration to save its life.[20]

Natural remedies usually do not provoke serious side effects. A physician shared this natural sinus remedy with me: Transfer some liquid chlorophyll from a large bottle (from health stores) to a small dropper bottle. Dilute with water to prevent stinging. Use one or more drops in each nostril at night before retiring for infection and nasal congestion. Chlorophyll is absolutely safe, since it is taken from green plant sources, mainly alfalfa. It is a specific for infections.

There are some nondrug inhalants which are blessedly helpful in dissolving mucus. One of these is a combination of several volatile oils including eucalyptus, peppermint, cajuput, juniper, wintergreen and clove oils plus menthol. It is called Olbas oil. This is a natural product from Switzerland, available in this country. A few drops can be added to a vaporizer to produce a mist for inhaling. It also comes in a small dry pocket inhalator for emergencies.[21]

Salt also is known to dissolve mucus (have you ever tried pouring salt on a garden slug, largely mucus, and slime, and watched it dissolve)? Add diluted sea salt to your vaporizer to produce a salt mist for inhalation to help dissolve mucus. You might ask your doctor about the oxygenated salt inhalation therapy given to a former U.S. president when he was hospitalized for a lung ailment. Glycothymoline, or even Tincture of Benzoin (both from drug stores) have relieved respiratory stuffiness when added to a room vaporizer. If you have one of those facial saunas, so popular in past years but now unavailable, get it out and use it as a vaporizer. I add whichever remedy I wish to the water, for inhalation purposes to help dissolve mucus.

You can make your own inhaler. Take a large empty juice can. Boil several inches of water in it, then remove from heat. Add a few drops of a mucus-dissolving inhalant[21] on the surface of the water and immediately cover it with a small tent made of a piece of typing paper, fastened on the side with a paper clip or tape, leaving a small hole at the top. Put a towel over your head and inhale this vapor for ten minutes. This remedy was suggested by William A. McGarey, M.D.

A nutritionist told me of another surprising remedy which worked for a man with severe emphysema. The man had not been able to walk more than a few steps. The remedy which reversed his problem was as follows: Five drops of anise oil (from drug stores) put on top of a small amount of brown sugar or honey in a small spoon, taken orally, thirty minutes before meals. The man reported to the nutritionist that, as a result, he was able to walk without any shortness of breath or other respiratory difficulty while climbing and walking at 7,000 feet in altitude, during a fishing vacation.

A remedy for asthma which sounds amusing is worth a try. Lay very thin slices of raw onion on a plate. Spread honey on each, cover with an inverted plate and let stand all night. From the syrup which results, take a teaspoon four times daily. The author, J. H. Oliver, says "it works like magic!"[22]

Dr. Marsh Morrison reports a natural treatment for asthmatic attacks. He learned that cranberries contain an ingredient which dilates bronchial tubes and helps normal breathing to become re-established. His formula: cook and mash raw unsweetened cranberries to a pulp. Refrigerate. When an asthmatic attack occurs, Dr. Morrison, says, mix a teaspoon or two of the cranberry pulp in a cup of warm water, and sip.

The Schuessler cell salts also promise help for respiratory ailments. Dr. Schuessler believed that asthma could result from a deficiency of certain minerals salts, which are found in the tiny homeopathic cell salt tablets, available from all homeopathic pharmacies and some health stores. They are dissolved dry on the tongue, according to directions on the label. One of these salts known as *Kali. Phos.* is said to bring relief in most cases. Another, *Kali. Mur.*, has also proved effective. One physician reported the case of a patient who was a chronic asthmatic. During an attack, the doctor gave the patient *Kali. Mur.* every twenty minutes until relieved of the attack, then every three hours. The patient later reported to the doctor that he had not had an attack since.[23]

A homeopathic physician will have further remedies to suggest. Such practitioners are rare in this country, though they are the rule in Europe. Even Queen Elizabeth maintains one permanently on her staff of health advisors. To find the name of one in your area, write to The National Center of Homeopathy, Suite 506, 6231 Leesburg Pike, Falls Church, Virginia, 22044.

Breathing Exercises

Certain breathing exercises are helpful for getting rid of old air and/or phlegm. Overbreathing excess air may complicate the problem. Inhaling in short gasps, rather than slow deep breaths may be preferable. One doctor has treated 400 asthmatics successfully by getting their heads lower than their feet, by putting the head on the hands on the floor while resting the feet on a bed or chair, in an upside-down position.[22]

The object of the following exercises is to slow down your rate of breathing so that you no longer have to pant; also to help the lungs to *exhale,* a difficult task when they are afflicted:

One simple remedy which you can use anywhere, any time, is the whistle exercise. You merely purse your lips as if you were going to whistle and exhale as slowly as possible. This can be done on the street, when you are climbing stairs—at *any* time, and no one will even notice.

At home you can do abdominal breathing. This exercise strengthens your lungs muscles and helps them exhale more easily. Lie on your back, knees bent. Inhale slowly, at the same time push out your stomach so that it protrudes. When you have inhaled as much air as possible and pushed your stomach out so that it protrudes as much as possible, *then* exhale by using the whistle exercise. Purse your lips and exhale very slowly. As Theodore Berland and Gordon Snider say in their helpful book, *Living With Your Bronchitis and Emphysema,* you do not have to think of your chest at all. "Concentrate only on the muscles of your abdomen, on its protruding as you inhale, on its squeezing tighter as you exhale. It may be helpful to repeat, even out loud, 'Breathe in, Belly out, Breathe out, Belly in.'"[12] You will find other helpful hints in this book. For example, to make sure you are strengthening your abdomen, you can put some heavy books on your stomach and literally push them upward as you make your abdomen protrude.

J. Frank Hurdle, M.D., gives a simple exercise he has found helpful in emphysema. He says, "It consists simply of spending five minutes, three times a day, blowing up balloons!" He recommends the thick type of balloon which really makes you red in the face to blow up. (This, of course, helps you to breathe OUT as we have found necessary for emphysema patients.) After this becomes comfortable during a period of two months, Dr. Hurdle increases the time blowing balloons to fifteen minutes three times a day. Since this increases tolerance to other exercise, Dr. Hurdle recommends gradual increase of exercise through calisthenics, hiking and eventually jogging. Patients have by this method overcome their emphysema and can exercise hard without becoming winded, he says.[24]

REFERENCES
(See *Bibliography* for fuller details.)

1. *The American Review of Respiratory Diseases*, September, 1972.
2. *United Press Report*, July 16, 1973.
3. Cleeland Bean, "Protect Yourself from Polluted Air," *Here's Health*, May, 1973.
4. Mike Samuels, M.D. and Hal Bennett, *The Well Body Book*.
5. J. I. Rodale and Staff, *The Encyclopedia of Common Diseases*.
6. "Warning on Asthma and Aspirin," *Associated Press* release, August 8, 1972.
7. *New England Journal of Medicine*, February 12, 1970.
8. Personal Communication. Also *Prevention*, June, 1970.
9. *The Journal of Asthma Research*, Vol. 9, No. 2, December, 1971. Carl J. Reich, M.D. Address: 2051 Medical Centre, Calgary 2, Alberta, Canada.

10. Ernest J. Sternglass, *Low Level Radiation*.
11. Linda Clark, *Are You Radioactive? How to Protect Yourself*.
12. Theodore Berland M.D. and Gordon L. Snider, M.D., *Living With Your Bronchitis and Emphysema*.
13. John J. Miller, Ph.D., "Vitamin E and Smog," *Journal of Applied Nutrition*, Vol. 23, Nos. 3 and 4, Winter, 1971.
14. *Chemical and Engineering News*, June 29, 1972.
15. Bicknell and Prescott, *The Vitamins in Medicine*.
16. Irwin Stone, *The Healing Factor, Vitamin C Against Disease*.
17. Linda Clark, *Get Well Naturally*.
18. "Try Vitamin E for Hay Fever," *Prevention*, August, 1973.
19. *The Medical Journal of Australia*, April 2, 1966.
20. *The German Medical Monthly*, April, 1959.
21. For information write Penn Herb Co., Ltd., 603 North 2nd St., Philadelphia, Pa. 19123.
22. J. H. Oliver, *Proven Remedies*.
23. J. B. Chapman, M.D., *Dr. Schuessler's Biochemistry*, (This wonderful little book is available at most homeopathic pharmacies in America.)
24. J. Frank Hurdle, M.D., *Doctor Hurdle's Program to Retain Youthfulness*.

7: BACKACHES

Backaches tend to be the rule, rather than the exception these days. According to research, I found that the major causes appear to be poor nutrition and a minimum of exercise.

Our forefathers, except for an occasional bout of lumbago or rheumatism, rarely complained of backaches. Today, unlike our antecedents, the average person is both nutritionally impoverished and underexercised. Our grandfathers and great-grandfathers did their own chores, planting, digging, pushed their own plows, sawed their own wood and walked or rode horseback (an exercise in itself), reserving a horse-and-buggy for long distance traveling or going to church on Sundays.

Our grandmothers, without labor saving appliances, built their own wood stove fires, beat the rugs without help from a vacuum cleaner, kneaded their own bread (another exercise in itself), filled and emptied the washtubs by hand, and made a lovely rub-a-dub-dub sound on an old-fashioned washboard. I know, because I watched these activities when I visited my own grandparents.

My grandfather was not a farmer, but a banker and an architect. He owned a car but he never used it except on Sundays. Otherwise he walked to work, twice daily, a two-mile distance each way, in the small, mile-high town in Colorado where they lived. He also pushed his own hand-driven lawnmower and shoveled his own snow.

My grandmother did not suffer from lack of women's lib, even though she did lack push-button appliances. She used organic food from farms or from her own garden, fertile eggs from her chickens and raw milk from her backyard cow, all of which she tended herself. She remained serene. Every afternoon by two o'clock, after dinner (the main meal—supper came in the evening), the dishes had been hand washed, the house was shining, and the blinds were drawn against the afternoon sun. She then took a nap before calling on her friends, attending social gatherings, a church auxiliary, visiting the sick, or whatever.

Yet, *never* in their lifetime, did I ever hear a complaint from either grandparent about a backache!

Today the average person is not only malnourished, but never stands when he can sit, walks when he can ride; and backaches are common.

Beside poor nutrition and lack of exercise, there are other minor causes of backache, too. They include:

Wrong types of beds or chairs that do not support the spine properly.

High or platform heels, which throw the spine and posture out of alignment. (The spine is a flexible hinge but it cannot take continuous strain or torture without eventually rebelling.)

Mechanical problems such as one shorter leg, a condition which can be remedied.

Strain, stress due to long sitting or improper lifting.

Injury, or acute or chronic disease such as kidney trouble, women's complaints, prostate problems, influenza or arthritis (covered in a previous chapter).

Even emotional problems can cause a backache; stiffness or painful cramping can result from tension.

Poor posture including a tipped pelvis and swayback, common in men and women.

The question, of course, is what to do about your backache. It can almost always be helped and often sooner than you think. The first thing is to relieve the pain. The next thing is to find the cause and eliminate it so that the pain will not return.

The first thing I would do if I had a backache would be to get to a chiropractor or osteopath as fast as possible. You can try a dog collar or use the traction route, even for a whiplash or other spinal disturbance, if you wish, but I would try a chiropractor or osteopath first. Even if such an injury is present, such a therapist can take an X-ray and establish the cause of the trouble. In lesser disturbances, the back pain can often be relieved in minutes.

A friend phoned to ask if there were any help available for "sacroiliac trouble" which can cause excruciating pain from hip to toe. She said she had had this pain for three months, could not find a comfortable sleeping position and someone had suggested it might be due to a sacroiliac problem. That "someone" made the diagnosis, not I, but it later turned out to be correct. Whatever the cause, I suggested a spinal adjustment and fast. My friend said she had never darkened the door of any but an M.D., but she was willing to try. So she gathered up her courage and went.

An hour later she called and said, "I can't believe it. That pain I was suffering from for three months disappeared within three minutes!"

This woman is well nourished and the cause had evidently been due to lifting a heavy rock in her garden. Later, she forgot her lesson, lifted another rock with the same result. Her sacroiliac responded as quickly to chiropractic treatment the second time, and from then on she left rock lifting to someone with a stronger back.

Men too often do not lift correctly. They should put the burden straight ahead of them, bend their knees, keep their spine straight, lift with their arms, then transfer the weight to their legs rather than their backs. If two people are lifting something together, they should agree to cooperate at the *same minute*, otherwise one gets most of the weight and the strain. And if you move furniture by yourself, lean against it and shove; don't push it with your arms. And do it slowly.

Using the wrong furniture can often cause a chronic backache. A chair that is too deep, or too short in the seat, making you curl up like a pretzel to try to fit it, doesn't help backs. Neither does the use of a stove, table or counter that is too low. If you cannot change their heights, get a stool which is the correct height for sitting at your work. This applies to typists, too. A desk, or chair, should be gauged to *your* measurements to avoid continuous bending. If your back aches from stooping in your garden, try kneeling.

Housewives should watch their carrying. Laundry baskets, babies, or large bags of groceries, should not be carried on one side only, causing one always to lean sideways. Keep the spine as straight as possible. And forget those high heels, platforms included. They not only distort the appearance, but the posture and spine as well. Many women are learning about the luxury of comfortable sandals or flats instead of looking ridiculous tottering about on stiletto heels or platforms.

One woman recently tripped herself up on her platform heels and acquired a seriously sprained ankle, which might have broken. Doctors say such accidents are happening widely as a result of wearing such shoes.

If you wonder if one leg is temporarily longer, lie on the floor and note whether your feet touch each other in perfect alignment. If not, a spinal adjustment may quickly solve the problem. I once took my limping mother to a chiropractor and saw for myself that one leg was one inch longer than the other. After an adjustment, which took minutes, both legs were equal and she glided out of the office.

If a person has a deformity of a permanent nature in which one leg is definitely shorter, an orthopedist can order a built-up shoe for the shorter leg.

Many people wake up tired and though they know it may be

due to an oversoft bed, they do nothing about it except to continue to suffer from fatigue. W. B. Parsons, M.D.[1] tells of a woman who went on a camping trip where she had to sleep on hard ground for many nights. She recovered from a backache which had plagued her for years. If your mattress and springs "give" too much and you cannot afford another set, make or buy a firm bed board to place between the mattress and springs. Otherwise treat yourself to a new bed which is firm enough so that your spine does not sag as you lie on it.

The Effect of Nutrition

Nutrition may provide help for your backache. In case you doubt this, stop a minute and think. It makes sense that even though a spinal manipulation can correct a misalignment, the spine may not be able to maintain this alignment if the muscles and tissues are weak or flabby. Too many carbohydrates and too little protein tend toward flabby muscles. For this reason, athletes are fed liberal amounts of protein and are restricted in carbohydrates. Even minerals are important for strengthening muscles. A friend has recurring problems with her axis and atlas, those two little bones at the top of the spine which are involved not only in good circulation to the head, eyes, ears and brain, but in controlling the alignment of the entire spine which lies below them. My friend always noted certain symptoms, usually vague discomfort without pain, when her axis and atlas were "out," always confirmed and adjusted by her chiropractor.

Recently she decided to clean out her garage. Having no help, she moved papers and shoved boxes herself and after she had finished the job, she decided to check with her chiropractor on the condition of her axis and atlas. To her own and the chiropractor's astonishment, in spite of her rugged activities, the atlas and axis had remained in place for the first time for several years. Her only change had been that she had added larger amounts of calcium to her diet. Different types of calcium are assimilated differently by various individuals, but whatever type I take, I always add some bone meal to support strong bones.

Other nutritional helps in keeping a back in place following spinal adjustments are Vitamin E and Manganese, both nutrients which have been found to strengthen muscles and ligaments.[2]

Incidentally, backache can be due to an allergy. John H. Tobe, of Canada, states that he suffered from backache for almost fifty years until he discovered that he was allergic to wheat and wheat products. When he gave these foods up, his backache disappeared. He states that others have found a similar reaction to wheat.

Adelle Davis states that over four million people in the U.S. suffer from severe backache due to abnormal or honeycombed bones, a result of too little calcium, magnesium and Vitamin D. She says, "When the diet is made adequate, particularly in protein, calcium, magnesium and vitamins C and D ... backaches and other symptoms usually disappear."[3]

Vitamin C alone has proved beneficial for low back pains. James Greenwood, Jr., M.D., of Baylor University College of Medicine, has found that using frequent doses of 500 to 1,000 mg. of Vitamin C (ascorbic acid) orally has relieved low back pain. He has also successfully treated more than 500 patients with slipped disc, including himself, with Vitamin C therapy.[4]

Pain in the sciatic nerve has yielded to continuous Vitamin B therapy.

Another surprising help for various forms of backaches comes from the Schuessler homeopathic cell salts, those minerals which come in tiny sweet pellets to be dissolved dry on the tongue, not gulped down with water. There are twelve salts, or minerals, and a deficiency of certain ones are related to different types of ailments, including backaches, as described in a book: *Dr. Schuessler's Biochemistry*, by J. B. Chapman, M.D. The book, as well as the salts themselves, are usually available from homeopathic pharmacies. If you cannot locate one of these stores in your area, write for information to Standard Homeopathic Pharmacy, P.O. Box 61067, Los Angeles, 90061.

One of these cell salts, known as *Mag. Phos.* (an abbreviation for Magnesium Phosphate) is used for the type of back pain that comes in spasms. A friend of mine woke up one morning with these excruciating spasms, and before the day was over she was screaming with pain. A call to a homeopathic adviser started her on the use of *Mag. Phos.*, not in the small dosage indicated on the bottle, but because of the severity of the pain, a teaspoon at a time. By the next morning the pain had completely disappeared and did not return, although the patient was advised to watch in the future for possible oncoming symptoms and take the minimum dose in order to prevent another serious attack.

Another friend, who has had a lifetime of back trouble, including spinal nerve surgery, has suffered for years from repeated attacks of back pain spasms, especially when her spine was out of alignment as established by her physician who had previously been an osteopath. He usually gave her an adjustment, advised bed rest, and she eventually recovered. One time, however, she experienced an attack and nothing helped, neither daily adjustments nor staying in bed around the clock while suffering agonies. When she learned about *Mag. Phos.* and took it like the first woman I mentioned, her pain also began to recede at the end of the day. Due to large *Mag. Phos.* dosage, by the next morning she was out of bed and out of pain. Whether at home or while traveling, she now refuses to be without this remedy.

A woman doctor in her 80s, drives alone often to a city 1,000 miles distant from her home, for business purposes. She has two rules for relaxed and comfortable driving: she takes *Mag. Phos.* at regular intervals and stops often to relax and stretch. She is not troubled with back pain or fatigue, she says. Cell salts are a form of nutrition. They are not drugs. *Mag. Phos.* is an easily assimilated form of magnesium.

Exercises For Your Back

Meanwhile, some exercises can help your back.

Many specialists believe that most backaches are due to muscles that are too stiff or too weak to work normally. Weak abdominal muscles have been found to be one cause of chronic backaches. Physicians at Iowa State University College of Medicine, found that the following exercise relieves forty-two out of fifty-eight backache sufferers:

Lie flat on your back. Tuck your toes under the strap of a slant board, or under the side of a bed or sofa. Clasp your hands behind your neck. Sit up ten or twelve times daily.

Another abdominal muscle exercise was responsible for relief of low back pain in 889 patients. This exercise was tested at Madigan General Hospital, Tacoma, Washington. The exercise is a variation of the sit-ups mentioned above:

Keeping legs straight, raise your hips and knees to a 45° angle and sit up. It is hard to do, but the 889 patients who used it fifteen to twenty times daily, five days a week, attested to its success.

Dr. Hans Kraus of New York University supplies some tips for prevention of back trouble for those who must work in sedentary occupations:

Exercise a few minutes daily.

Change your chair from time to time.

Take five minute breaks for walking or stretching.

When driving long distances, stop often and relax.

Your neck can influence your back. Neck tension is common these days, due to driving a car as well as doing desk or other concentrated work. One of the best known exercises is to sit down and, stretching your neck to full capacity, roll it in a wide circle, first to the far right, then backward, then to the far left, and finally down to your check. Repeat three times clockwise, then three times counterclockwise.

I would like to share another exercise I learned recently from a physiotherapist who told me it could relieve not only neck tension, but help realign the atlas and axis. The physiotherapist assured me that the exercise is safe for anyone at any time. Here it is:

Pull a chair up to the side of your bed. Sit straight in the chair. Stretch your legs straight in front of you on the bed, palms of your hands resting on your knees. Now drop your head so that it hangs heavy by its *full* weight against your chest. You should feel a definite stretch at the back of your neck. Remain in this position for ten minutes. Those who have tried it report that the after-effects are "great."

One of the most exciting exercises I have learned about recently is Dr. Alec Thompson's do-it-yourself exercise for displaced sacroiliac. Many people have bent over to pick up something when, with a sharp pain, their back "went out" and they were "frozen," unable to move. If a chiropractor or osteopath is handy, the adjustment can be made quickly. If not, you are in trouble as well as in agony. Dr. Thompson's exercise which he has taught to all of his patients ends all of this needless suffering. There is much more information in the fascinating book about Dr. Thompson, written by Jess Stearn, showing how a slipped sacroiliac, though possibly unnoticed, has caused all sorts of disturbances throughout the body. Even a swollen thumb has responded, once the sacroiliac has been set right by this exercise. I heartily encourage you to read the book for yourself, but I will try to explain the simple self-help exercise by which you can put in your own sacroiliac. Just a few days ago I lent my copy of this book to a friend who is prone to back troubles. She has her favorite osteopath on whom she relies whenever her back becomes misaligned, and when I offered to lend her the book, she said, "I have had back trouble so long that I know all the exercises and all the tricks to handle my back." But I loaned it to her anyway.

Several days later she called and said, "Well, Dr. Thompson's exercise saved me from untold suffering. Over the weekend [when her osteopath's office was closed] I leaned over, and snap, went my back! I didn't think I would ever be able to move again. I couldn't even crawl to the telephone for help. But I did ease myself to the floor and did the exercise. My back went back into place and I have had no pain or trouble since. I worked in my garden all the rest of the day."

Here is the exercise. Lie down, back flat on the floor. Bend your right knee outward grasp it with your right hand, pulling it toward your head as far as possible. Your heel should automatically be touching your groin. Hold it! Now grasp your right ankle with your left hand, and using both hands, pull your ankle and knee toward your shoulder, trying to press down both knee and ankle simultaneously against your body. Hold to a count of thirty seconds or as long as you can stand it. Then slowly release your knee and ankle, and lay your right leg on the floor. As you do, if your sacroiliac is "out" on that side, you will feel a click, meaning that it has gone into place.

Repeat with the left leg. The exercise is really easy and is harder to explain than to do. The Stearn book shows an illustration which makes it easier to understand. Many people I know do this exercise every night and morning for prevention purposes.[5]

So with common sense, good nutrition and proper exercise, you should be able to get your back into line. In turn it will keep you comfortable, a reward well worth your efforts.

REFERENCES
(See *Bibliography* for fuller details.)

1. *Canadian Medical Association Journal*, July, 1951.
2. J. Ronald Mikels, "Vitamin E and Manganese Help Your Back Stay Adjusted." *Prevention*, May, 1973.
3. Adelle Davis, *Let's Get Well*.
4. Linda Clark, *Get Well Naturally*.
5. Jess Stearn: *Dr. Thompson's New Way for You to Cure Your Aching Back*. (Excerpts used by permission.)

8: CANCER

I have previously covered cancer in my book, *Get Well Naturally*. Although published several years ago, little change has taken place in this field, despite the sharp rise in cancer cases.

According to Nobel Prizewinning biologist, James D. Watson, professor of molecular biology at Harvard, in spite of millions of dollars spent on a rapid increase of cancer treatment centers, the result is little actual understanding of cancer or real knowledge of how to treat it. Consequently, Dr. Watson considers the nation's cancer program a total sham.

He says, "The American public is being sold a nasty bill of goods about cancer. While they are being told about cancer cures, the cure rate has improved only about 1 per cent. The grim cancer statistics are about as bad as ever." *(Associated Press* release, March 7, 1975.)

The subject of cancer is still controversial. Orthodox medicine uses only radiation, chemotherapy and surgery for this disease.

There are other groups who believe that nontoxic cancer therapies should be allowed testing (so far denied) as well as use. Because many cancer patients prefer a nontoxic therapy, or other natural remedies, these groups have organized to provide such information for those who wish it. As the *Organic Consumer Report*, February 4, 1975, states, "The time has come, in fact is long past, when no one should overlook or ridicule *anything* demonstrated to be effective in reversing, controlling or preventing cancer."

The following groups exist as nonprofit, educational organizations which provide literature on natural cancer remedies, present lectures, conventions, and information from outstanding researchers and doctors on the subject of natural, safe, cancer treatment.

I am listing two of these courageous organizations which are sustained only by memberships and donations. You may write to one of your choice for information. I am listing them in alphabetical order:

Cancer Control Society

The Cancer Control Society is a nonprofit, educational, charitable organization dedicated to educating the public and professionals about promising nontoxic cancer therapies such as Laetrile (Vit. B-17) and measures taken in other nutritionally related diseases.

The functions of the Society consist of distributing free "Information Sets" with updated doctor and source lists of amygdalin (Vitamin B-17) and other therapies; publishing a bimonthly journal called *Cancer Control Journal*; maintaining a Cancer Book House; renting and distributing a historical documentary motion picture called "Nature's Answer to Cancer"; having an Annual Convention in September in Los Angeles, and encouraging more Chapters to form. Chapters are now located in Kalamazoo, Michigan; Las Vegas, Nevada, and Anaheim, California. The National Headquarters is located at: 2043 N. Berendo, Los Angeles, Calif. 90027. Telephone 213-663-7801.

The International Association of Cancer Victims and Friends, Inc.
This group:
Publishes the *Cancer News Journal* with articles by outstanding and well-known national and international experts in fields of medicine, nutrition, natural therapies, law and research.

Specializes in providing information to the people on a very wide variety of nontoxic cancer treatments, most of which are virtually unpublicized.

Stimulates interest of the layman and medical and allied professionals in the nontoxic, noninjurious approach in cancer and nutritional disorders.

Encourages impartial investigation by our governmental and private agencies of ALL hopeful cancer therapies and ALL possible cancer causes.

Fosters medical freedom of choice for doctor and patient.

Serves as a clearing house for the accumulation and distribution of literature.

The National Headquarters is located at: P.O. Box 707, 155 D. South Highway 101, Solana Beach, Calif. 92075. Telephone 714-755-9781. (A suburb of San Diego, California)

I.A.C.V.F. Chapters and Addresses:

ARIZONA:
Metro-Phoenix Chapter
P.O. Box 1541
Mesa, AZ 85201

Tucson Chapter
P.O. Box 27387
Tucson, AZ 85726
602-624-2441

CALIFORNIA:
Bay Area Chapter
593 Arkansas St.
San Francisco, Ca. 94107

Peninsula Chapter
P.O. Box 5081
San Mateo, Ca. 94402

San Jose—Santa Cruz Chapter
552 S. Bascom Avenue
San Jose, Ca. 95128
408-295-7242
408-379-0597

FLORIDA:
Central Florida Chapter
P.O. Box 6387
Orlando, FL 32803
305-671-4231

HAWAII:
Hawaii Chapter
3035 Kiele Avenue
Honolulu, HI 96815

ILLINOIS:
Chicago Chapter
P.O. Box 347
Riverside, IL 60546

MICHIGAN:
Southern Michigan Chapter
5350 S. Meridian Rd.
Jackson, MI 49201
517-787-5459

MINNESOTA:
Twin Cities Chapter
P.O. Box 8171
St. Paul, MN 55113
612-489-9479

NEW YORK:
Long Island, N. Y. Chapter
2787 Long Beach Rd.
Oceanside, N.Y. 11572
516-764-4666

New York City Chapter
464 Beach 145 Street
Rockaway Park, N.Y. 11694
212-634-2762
212-474-5392

TEXAS:
El Paso Chapter
3039 Wheeling Avenue
El Paso, Texas 79930
915-565-3103

WASHINGTON:
Bellevue Chapter
1004 Rosemont Blvd.
Bellevue, WA 98008
206-747-7107

There is a third source of help: a paperback book, *March of Truth on Cancer,* describes seventy-nine safe, natural and comparatively inexpensive cancer treatments and where they may be found. The book also provides other excellent information for cancer patients, supplying the *truth,* not biased opinions.

This book is on sale for $5.00 from The Arlin J. Brown Information Center, P.O. Box 251, Ft. Belvoir, Virginia 22060.

9: PREVENTION AND TREATMENT OF CATARACTS

There is a lack of understanding about cataracts. Most people believe a cataract is a cataract, so if there is a remedy available, it should work for all. This is not necessarily true. Many people write asking me to suggest a remedy. These letters are usually pitiful, like the one from a man who wrote:

"Please give me help for my cataracts. My doctor says surgery is the only solution, but I do not want to submit to the knife if there is any alternative.

"Meanwhile, I am in dire need of help since I am going blind and have four children who live with and depend upon me. I lost my wife several years ago. Although my sight wavers, I can see enough to shop and cook. Sometimes with glasses I can drive short distances, but not for long periods. I was a welder by trade, but the doctor told me to quit so I am on a pension. He has treated me for some time, but since nothing has helped, he finally said surgery was all that was left. I got so nervous when I was told this, I walked out of the office. Any suggestions you can give me will be more than appreciated. Yours respectfully, G.I."

There *is* help for many cataract sufferers, but what may help one person may not help another. I would give anything if I could pull a rabbit out of a hat and send this man, or anyone else, a sure-fire remedy. But even if I knew the right one for his particular case, I am not allowed to prescribe, suggest, or recommend *anything* concerning a medical problem, since this would be construed by the authorities as practicing medicine without a license. Fortunately, since we still have freedom of speech and the press, I can report research, together with the source where I learned the information, and share it with you so that you may choose, and use it as you wish.

Eye specialists have found that there are at least thirty-two types of cataracts, and at most over a hundred different varieties. Each type may call for a different kind of treatment. Unfortunately, many doctors do not know how to determine which type the patient may have and thus may not be able to pinpoint the specific remedy. Some types of cataract are due to calcium or other mineral deposits, or a combination of any of these. Thus what may work for one type might be useless for another.

John J. Miller, Ph.D. lists ten major causes of cataracts, resulting from his research-in-depth on this ailment:

1.–Galactose in excess (from milk)
2.–Glutathine deficiency
3.–Mineral and enzyme imbalance
4.–Hyperglycemia and diabetes
5.–Vitamin deficiencies, especially Vitamin C
6.–Amino acid deficiencies and imbalances (amino acids occur in proteins).
7.–Fatty acid intolerances. Half of the total fats in the eyes are unsaturated.
8.–Alloxan synthesis
9.–Aging
10.–Irradiation and drugs.

To complicate the situation, cataracts are currently reaching an all-time high, becoming almost epidemic. Possible, even probable, reasons for this sudden proliferation will be discussed later.

Not only is the *type* of cataract a factor in treatment, but the *stage* of its development, is involved. A cataract caught early, may be easier to reverse than one which is "ripe" enough for surgery. To be honest, there are some types for which no known alternative is known. But there are also cases in which a reprieve has appeared at the last moment, and the sight has been saved by a nonsurgical method. Since doctors usually recommend waiting several years for the cataract to ripen so that surgery can be performed, there is time to try one of the safe, natural remedies in the interim while waiting for the deadline, and without fear of causing further complications. Obviously, prevention is the best method of all. At the first sign of any unusual vision disturbance, immediate action is suggested.

In one eye clinic in the Southeastern U.S., ophthalmologists are using an electronic miscroscope, together with the analysis of the patient's molecular chemistry, to help identify the type of cataract, as well as the cause. The identification may, or may not, also determine the right treatment. Until other ophthalmologists employ this method, if you have had a reliable diagnosis of cataract by an eye specialist, perhaps by your own trial and error, your guess and use of a safe and natural remedy might be as good as the next person's. Date the diagnosis and check-ups to see if the method is working.

Here is an example from an intelligent woman, whose eye specialist diagnosed her cataract, but did not know the type or what to recommend, other than waiting for the ripening process at which time surgery could be used. He was willing, in the meantime, to let the woman experiment with safe, natural remedies and report what he found. She sent the following report to me:

Jan., 1973: My eye specialist found some improvement in my cataract. He also found that it had changed in shape from a Christmas tree to a figure 8. (Cataracts can come in all shapes.) Thus far, I have not been able to detect any improvement in vision.

April, 1973: My eye specialist has still not been able to determine the exact type of cataract. [No further report given.]

Sept., 1973: I have been under terrific emotional stress since my last check-up, supposed to affect cataracts, but my eye specialist found more improvement in my cataract in spite of everything.

Naturally you are interested in what this woman was doing, even though the treatment might not apply to you. In general, she had made a change in her diet, and used some natural substances in her eyes, about which I will tell you later.

What Is A Cataract?

Ophthalmologists may shudder at the nontechnical definitions which follow, but I am giving you explanations the average person can understand. If they do not satisfy you, I suggest that you stop in the nearest library and look up the definition of the many types of cataracts in a medical dictionary. There are forty-nine kinds listed in my medical dictionary, all described in technical terms. The simplest is "Opacity of the crystalline lens or its capsule." Even experts do not always agree. Some say that a cataract is not a growth but a gradual loss of transparency in the eye lens, producing a loss of vision according to the extent and location of the cataract. Another version is that one form of cataract is a skin or film forming over the eyeball, whereas another form is a cyst which grows into the eye itself. In other words, one type only covers and irritates the retina, whereas the other type attaches itself more deeply. Still another explanation is that a cataract is made up of dead cells which resemble fish scales accumulating in layers on the eye, resulting in opacity. John H. Tobe, in his book on cataracts,[1] believes that there are two main types: "developmental" or "degenerative." The developmental variety, he explains, occurs as a result of heredity, inflammatory or nutritional disturbances, whereas the degenerative type, with a gradual loss of transparency, results from degenerative changes.

Still another type results from exposure to continuous ultraviolet rays, as well as to great or continuous heat, including infrared rays. Dogs that sleep before, or stare at, a fireplace fire often develop cataracts. And there is evidence that exposure to leaking microwave ovens or radar, can apparently coagulate or "cook" the protein fraction in the lens of the eye.[2] Obviously such serious types of cataracts may be irreversible; so prevention is imperative.

What Causes Cataracts?

1. Although a cataract may seem to be a local eye problem, one ophthalmologist, who has treated cataracts successfully for many years, believes that it reflects an ailment in the body such as a toxic condition, gastrointestinal, gastroenteritic, gall bladder disturbance, etc. Cataracts associated with diabetes have long been recognized. There is much confirmation of the correlation of poor health and cataracts. An eye specialist in England has written to me that liver ailments, hormone imbalance, and chronic or debilitating illnesses play an important part in the development of both cataract and glaucoma. He adds, "The transparency of the crystalline lens is maintained by the flow of the aqueous, a watery fluid precipitated from the bloodstream. Should this flow become too slow, the lens is insufficiently 'fed' and it begins to resemble a dirty window. Later, as the condition develops, definite opacities form and disturb the vision. When illness of the body cause impurities in the blood, the aqueous may also be affected and different types of cataracts commence to develop."[3]

The late Dr. Royal Lee believed that cataract could be caused by direct trauma (injury to the eye), toxemia, X-rays, inflammatory disturbances and heredity, or in association with diabetes, arteriosclerosis, hypothyroid, hypercholesterol and malnutrition.

Remember that the eyes, as well as ears, teeth, and head are not separate entities, but a continuation of the body. To have good eye health, you must have good body health.

2. Cataracts are sometimes the result of too much, or too little of a substance in the body. This may be because the body is fed too little of a certain nutrient (i.e., calcium, or protein), or on ac-

count of faulty body metabolism, it may not assimilate properly the substances which already are present. We are learning that arthritis may be due to unassimilated calcium which may pile up in the joints or elsewhere in the body instead of being kept in solution. Some cataracts are similarly due to excessive calcium or other mineral deposits in the eyes. Dr. Melvin E. Page characterizes these as "arthritis of the eye." Lack of hydrochloric acid, needed to dissolve calcium within the body, may also be a cause. Apple cider vinegar may help here. Protein, as well as calcium, also needs acid for its assimilation.

3. Slowed circulation, preventing the proper nutrients from reaching the eyes, is also a problem in many cataracts. This does not mean circulation of the blood only, but the proper lymph flow to provide drainage and elimination of body toxins to allow absorption of cataracts. Again and again the Edgar Cayce readings advise osteopathic manipulations of the cervical and upper dorsal areas of the cerebro-spinal system to relieve congestion and facilitate the circulation to and from the eyes.

4. Some drugs and chemicals, too numerous to list here, have caused cataracts. Usually these drugs have been prescribed in conditions, such as reducing, and produced cataracts as a side effect. In some instances, after a long expensive battle in which the patient has sued the drug company, he has won; in others he has lost. John Tobe points an accusing finger at nitrates and nitrites, additives allowed in bacon, ham, hot dogs and luncheon meats (cold cuts).

Another substance involved in cataracts is sorbitol, a food additive which is both a chemical to provide sweetening as well as moisture in shredded coconut, marshmallows, some confections, and other food products. Sorbitol strongly aggravates cataracts in animals, so read your labels and avoid it.[4]

One drug which was formerly thought to be a cause of cataracts has been exonerated: DMSO (dimethyl sulfoxide). Stanley W. Jacob, M.D. of the University of Oregon Medical School, and a pioneer researcher on DMSO says, "It is true that in some lower species of laboratory animals a change in the refractive index of the lens, *not a true cataract,* develops with large doses of DMSO. The best informed scientific opinion has concluded that this does not occur in monkeys. Careful, long term follow-up has shown that this does not occur in man."

5. Radiation, or radioactivity, is now found to be a factor in many cataracts, as shown in my book, *Are You Radioactive: How to Protect Yourself.*[2] Not only is radioactivity a by-product of nuclear fall-out from detonated bombs, but of radiation from fluorescent lights, television (watching for prolonged periods, especially color TV) as well as exposure to radar and leaking microwave ovens and towers. Various forms of nuclear exposure have been incriminated in cataract development by some air force doctors, and cautiously admitted by some government bulletins. Some air force veterans are charging that their cataracts are the result of exposure to radar.[2,5] Nuclear plants can also be a factor.[2] In these cases, which may not be reversible, the best remedy is to avoid exposure *before* cataracts begin!

6. Stress, which may interfere with the body's circulation system, is one of the most common causes of all. Many years ago, one therapist who uses the Bates method of relaxation for vision problems, said that he had found in every case of cataract that the patient had previously suffered from some form of prolonged stress or sudden shock. Even though this predated our nuclear problem, the effect still stands. Adelle Davis told the story of the woman who repeatedly was taken by her husband, a mining engineer, into areas far from the comforts of civilization, on field trips which she hated. She repeatedly developed cataracts in both eyes, which disappeared when she returned to New York City, which she loved.[6]

I recently heard of a woman who lost her husband upon whom she had leaned heavily for solutions to problems large and small. After his death, she found it necessary to make her own decisions, which she considered intolerable and almost impossible. Her vision began to dim and one doctor diagnosed her condition as cataracts, warning her that surgery was imminent. She was urged by a friend to seek a second opinion from another doctor. He learned of her domestic plight and said he found no sign of cataracts, merely a temporary interference with her vision. Sure enough, as the woman gradually learned to become independent and felt more secure in leaning upon herself, her eye condition disappeared entirely. Her problem had been caused by severe and continuous stress and strain which had lasted for over a year.

7. The most obvious cause of many cataracts seems to be poor nutrition. This may even be the explanation of the type of cataract commonly called senile or aging cataract. The cause may be a lifetime of malnutrition coupled with poor circulation, also common in older people.

John H. Tobe writes, "From the information that I have accumulated, it would appear that the eyes are the mirror of what goes on inside your body . . . the way I look at it, in cataract, the eye is poorly nourished. The supply route is bad or failing and the eye is grossly undernourished. Basically it lacks the ability to feed and drain itself."[1]

This concept is confirmed by many specialists.

Morgan B. Raiford, M.D., ophthalmologist, has been studying cataracts for many years, both in the private clinic in Georgia, with which he is associated, and with colleagues at Georgia Institute of Technology. Dr. Raiford holds the opinion that faulty nutrition is a basic factor in cataract, and he has found that prevention of cataract is initiated by improving nutrition and body chemistry. For example, there are millions of people in India and Pakistan, he reports, who are suffering from "sugar cataracts" in their late 30's and 40's, due to a low-protein, high-carbohydrate diet. Dr. Raiford and his staff are cooperating with Dr. Kirmani, of the Jinnah Post-graduate Medical Centre, Karachi, Pakistan, trying to find out how the sugar changes in relation to the eye can be eliminated.

Dr. Donald T. Atkinson agrees with Dr. Raiford and others that cataracts can result from poor nutrition, resulting in lack of proper nourishment to the eye, after learning that cataract patients living in his area had one factor in common: poor, devitalized diets. He put 450 patients on a diet of eight to ten glasses of water, garden greens, a pint of milk (at least), two eggs and Vitamins A and C daily. He reports that he was successful in preventing cataracts in all 450 patients on this diet.[7]

Since government studies have found that many people are nutritionally impoverished in the United States, this, added to the radioactivity threat, may explain why cataracts are increasing so rapidly.

There has been a great controversy about whether or not milk products can cause cataracts. One explanation has been given by Dr. Ernest Beutler, a geneticist at the City of Hope Hospital in Los Angeles, to the effect that children and young adults who have cataracts may have an inherited metabolic defect which prevents them from assimilating milk properly. When this defect was found in children, they were put on a milk-free diet.

However, there is another explanation advanced by several other researchers. This is the theory that children in underprivileged countries, who cannot get milk after weaning, lose the ability to digest it because an enzyme, *lactase*, needed to assimilate *lactose* (a milk sugar) becomes deficient in the body, leading to lack of tolerance of lactose or galactose, found in milk. This, in turn, may lead to cataracts and may also affect many adults in the U.S. and elsewhere. This was found to be the case in the widely publicized Johns Hopkins rats which developed cataracts on an all-yogurt diet. It was not apparently learned until later that rats do not naturally manufacture lactase, thus could not metabolize the galactose in the yogurt. And still more important, it was learned that galactose, an ingredient of milk and milk products, is an antagonist to Vitamin B-2, the lack of which may play a part in cataract formation.

Adelle Davis stated that every type of animal studied, including fish and geese, developed cataracts when deprived of vitamin B-2 or riboflavin, Dr. P. S. Day, of Columbia University, found that a lack of Vitamin B-2 can cause cataracts in both animals and humans.[8] And Dr. Lewis Sydenstricker, of the University of Georgia Hospital, treated many cases of opacities with 15 mg. of B-2 daily, and though it took nine months, he reported that the opacities were reversed. If the Vitamin B-2 diet were stopped, the cataracts reappeared.[9]

However, if there is a deficiency of this vitamin, there are other B-2 deficiency symptoms which will appear before the cataract: a feeling of sand under the eyelids, cracks at the corners of the mouth, scaling around the nose, a purplish tongue, and others.[6,10]

The effect of galactose is not a simple problem, but is becoming more complex with time and continued research. It is complicated by today's step-up in milk products. John J. Miller, Ph.D., who has done extensive research on the cataract problem, says, "When milk was produced by the family cow for our ancestors, and used as a whole unmodified food, the problem was not so serious. But through development of the cheese industry, the promotion of yogurt, the evaporated milk program, and the powdered milk business, the concentration of galactose in our daily diet has been markedly increased."[11]

When there is a dietary excess of galactose, which has led to cataracts in the lens of the eyes of rats, a galactose-free diet may stop the trend toward cataract development by restoring lens fibers.[12] The problem may not be as great for those who can metabolize galactose, but for those who cannot, either riboflavin (Vitamin B-2) or orotic acid (another B vitamin), or perhaps both, have been found to be natural nutrients for improving galactose metabolism.

Vitamin B-2 is not the only vitamin deficiency involved in cataracts. Animals can develop cataracts due to lack of Vitamins E, D, pantothenic acid (a B vitamin), and tryptophane, a protein factor or amino acid which requires Vitamin B-6 for assimilation.[6] Vitamin C is also involved. Studies in India show that the cataractous eye has a lower content of ascorbic acid (Vitamin C) than normal eyes.[13]

Now that you have been given a glimpse into the causal problems involved in treating cataracts, let's turn to the exciting reports in which cataracts have been actually reversed, as well as remedies which have been found helpful.

Natural Treatments

One therapist recommends the Bates method for relaxation of the eyes since she believes that in addition to reflecting body disturbances, the eyes may also reflect a form of stress or psychosomatic condition.[14] There are many books written about the Bates method of eye training and relaxation. The book this therapist recommends is *Relax and See*, by Clara A. Hackett and Lawrence Galton, with a foreword by William Gutman, M.D. Dr. Gutman says, "I have seen excellent results of this system of eye training, even where severe pathology was present."[15]

Miss Hackett has worked successfully with 2,800 patients suffering from all manner of eye troubles: dimming vision, nearsightedness, farsightedness, cataracts and glaucoma. She has been responsible for improving vision, sometimes within a few weeks. There are case histories in the book of the recovery of cataract (and glaucoma) with the exact procedure to follow, described clearly. This book has been out of print for several years, but is now available. It is published in England by Faber and Faber, 24 Russell Square, London, and can be ordered through your bookstore.

Another therapist who has specialized in the Bates method in the U.S., found that over 90% of the cataract patients who used the system under supervision attained the following effects:

1.–The cataracts stopped developing.

2.–The cataracts were reduced and the vision improved on a continuing basis.

3.–The need for surgery was eliminated.

4.–Tension was involved in the majority of patients seen; thus correct eye relaxation helped to reverse the condition.

In addition to recommendation of osteopathic manipulations in the cervical and upper dorsal regions of the spine to relieve congestion, the Edgar Cayce readings advised certain head and neck exercises to be used morning and night, *every day*. In fact, in information given on cataracts, the readings cautioned the person afflicted to be patient, persistent, and consistent for at least six months if good results were desired.[16] This good advice applies to any of the other remedies I have mentioned, too.

The Cayce exercises are as follows: In a seated position, bend your head with neck fully stretched, forward three times, backward three times, to the right shoulder three times and to the left shoulder three times. Then circle, with neck at full stretch, clockwise to the right three times, then counterclockwise to the left, three times. Jess Stearn reports some surprising and excellent results with vision improvement in general from these exercises.[17]

Natural outdoor light has also been found necessary to aid good vision. Dr. John Ott points out that animals and people continually subjected to darkness or artificial light have developed dim vision. He even frowns on dark glasses for constant use.[18]

Perhaps the most astounding method of treating cataracts of all, is that of R. Brooks Simpkins, of England, who is a researcher and practitioner of eye problems through color therapy. He states in his book,[19] "Research has discovered that wave bands of color of the visible spectrum have individual and potent energic and medicinal properties which provide a natural medicine for the eyes and vision."

The effect of color therapy can be amazing, but not only the correct color should be chosen for the condition, but the correct *shade*. Each color has a certain frequency or vibration, and the *exact* frequency for the problem must be used, or it won't work. Ultraviolet and infrared rays, researchers feel, should not be used in any case due to their potential danger.

Mr. Simpkins has been using visible ray (color) therapy for eyes for over twenty-three years. He says, "I have found these rays to be efficacious in dispersing cataracts in many stages of development, in preventing such development, and also in preventing glaucoma from becoming chronic. These rays are also very helpful in the remedial treatment of affections such as choroiditis, iritis, retinitis, corneal opacities and con- junctivitis . . . help muscular imbalance of the eyes, and effec- tively help the recoordination of the retinae with visual centers of the brain."

Mr. Simpkins has developed a machine, called the *Fixoscope*. His patient is seated in a dark room at a table on which this machine rests and he peers through two openings, one for each eye, at the prescribed color which has been inserted between the eyes and a low intensity lamp, six inches away from the eyes. As a matter of fact, Mr. Simpkin's first model was nothing more than a flashlight for each eye containing two 2.4 volt flashlight bat- teries placed behind the color, six inches away from the eye of the viewer. The improved projector-like 12-volt, 12-watt illumi- nated machine into which the patient stares at the color chosen for his condition, has brought surprising results. Mr. Simpkins writes, "These visible rays give us a remedial therapy which no other method can be expected to achieve . . . in many patients who had been previously told that nothing more could be done for their eyes . . . during the last quarter of a century large numbers of people have been astonished at the improvement after even a single treatment."

Mr. Simpkins, in explaining the effect of the colors used for cataract, says, "We are all familiar with the properties of turpen- tine for thinning down paint which is too thick. The *correct* wavelength of green has a similar effect for congestive condi- tions in the eye, particularly in glaucoma. In all cases of glaucoma the green rays are of outstanding importance: the raised intraocular pressure usually goes down after a ten-minute exposure . . . such persons are given an intensified treatment in the form of two treatments daily, two times a week. The green rays are also used for dispersing cataractous conditions of the crystalline lens, for cloudy and 'frosted' corneal surfaces from previous ulceration. . . . "

Green is not the only helpful color. Red is also used for stimulation, and blue is used last in the treatment for a sedation effect. The Simpkins schedule for cataracts is as follows:

10 minutes red
10 minutes green
5 minutes blue

Mr. Simpkins states, "As cataractous conditions are broken down by the powerful red rays, as well as by the other less penetrating rays, the microscopic particles are apparently dissolved by the aqueous or conveyed by this fluid . . . for absorption into the blood stream. The absorption rate varies with the individual."

For those patients who live in or near England, one treatment of twenty-five minutes each, five days a week is sufficient and usually lasts a month. (The two day rest appears to be helpful.) For those who come from a distance for treatment, the treatments are used twice daily, at least three hours apart.

Unfortunately, authorities in the U.S. have banned all color therapy treatments, including the Simpkins *Fixoscope*, apparently because, though the treatments are far safer than questionable chemicals and drugs, they are competitive. Anyone who can get to England can write for an appointment to Mr. Simpkins (see references for his address).[20]

Many ask if after all, as the doctors insist, surgery is not the simplest solution to cataracts. This is a last resort only. I know two people well who have submitted to cataract surgery in both eyes. They get their driver's licenses and read without trouble. However, they are both definitely handicapped, because without their glasses they cannot see, and even with their glasses they have no side vision at all. Limited vision, of course, is better than none, but many who have had surgery deny that their vision is as "good as new."

According to George C. Thosteson, M.D., those who have had cataract surgery are more prone than others to retinal detachment and hemorrhaging. For this reason it is wise not to bump one's head or resume heavy work for at least two months following surgery. Even then, Dr. Thosteson warns, avoid straining, heavy lifting and a fall, which could be dangerous. Avoid ladders since it takes time for vision adjustment.

Other questionable methods of cataract removal, instead of the knife, are still in the experimental stage. One ophthalmologist who uses natural methods successfully told me that three patients had come to him who had submitted to the laser beam, which had not cleared the cataract effectively and had damaged the brain tissues, leaving the victim with a lifetime sentence of brain damage.

Again I issue a call for prevention, if possible, or at least a trial of natural remedies—which follow—although most doctors insist these cannot work. They *have* worked for some people and at least, being safe, are worth a try.

Natural Remedies

In listing the natural remedies, remember that I am not making claims. I am listing them because they have helped some people. The sources are often obscure, since in many cases they have been handed down generation by generation, either by word of mouth, or reprinted and copied in many books. Their sources are not considered scientific by orthodox practitioners, but who cares, if they work? Here are some natural remedies for cataracts that I have discovered in my research:

1.–One therapist suggests the use of castor oil in the eye. It is applied by dipping the finger in the castor oil bottle and smoothing it around the edge of the eye so that it can flow into the eye. If, after a month's trial there is no improvement, this therapist changes to linseed oil.

2.–Linseed oil can be applied by transferring some from the bottle obtained from the drug store (*not* the hardware store) to a sterile dropper bottle. One drop of linseed oil is put in the eye every night.

John Tobe, in his book, tells of a dog, nearly blind with cataracts, that regained normal sight after linseed oil therapy, and the cataracts were eliminated. The treatment was suggested by a veterinarian. Mr. Tobe also cites the case of a physician who, at the age of ninety, not only did not need glasses himself, but was well known for the successful treatment of cataracts of his patients, even those who had been warned that surgery would be eventually necessary. These patients had their sight restored, gave up their glasses and avoided surgery by linseed oil.[1]

3.–The late Charles Ahlson, an expert researcher on sea water, suggested (in addition to filtered sea water being added to the diets explained in another of my books[21]) the use of two or three drops of the filtered sea water (available from health stores, *not* from contaminated close-to-shore ocean water) in the eye night and morning.

Charles Perry, the English beauty expert, recommends sea water as an eyebath for tired, sore eyes.[22] You would think, being salty, that sea water would irritate the eyes, which it may for a few seconds only. But since tears contain salt, no damage can result from this natural saline solution. It is surprisingly restful and soothing to the eyes. I know, because I have tried it.

Dr. M. O. Garten in his book[23] tells of a doctor who had tried everything for his cataract except surgery, which had been advised. By taking sea water internally for nine months, he got rid of both a case of bursitis with which he had been afflicted for twenty years, *and* his cataract.

4.–Another folk remedy is that of a raw potato poultice. It is made of grated old potato without the skin, placed between two layers of gauze, and placed on the closed eyelid for an hour or more daily. The theory is that of most other types of poultices used for various conditions: a drawing out of toxic waste.

Other assorted natural remedies include a drop of fresh lemon juice or diluted apple cider vinegar (they both sting at first); the jelly from a piece of fresh cut aloe rubbed into the eye; fresh milk from a coconut, which may be kept for a few days in the refrigerator. The use of mashed fresh papaya, rubbed into the edge of the eye, has also been reported.

5.–Although she did not specifically mention any connection between the two, the late Claudia V. James may have unknowingly discovered an herbal treatment which *might* help dissolve at least one type of cataract. It is a special use of camomile tea.[24] I searched many herb books and learned that Culpeper wrote about camomile, "It most wonderfully breaketh the stone." Other herbal books recommended it for many things, including an eye wash.

The cooled camomile tea could be transferred to a clean dropper bottle obtained from a drug store, and perhaps used as an eye wash or as eye drops morning and night. At any rate, the herbalists consider it safe to put into the eyes, so it might be worth a try. Like any other natural treatment, don't give up too soon. (If you achieve any results, please let me know.)

6.–One of the most dramatic natural remedies is that of eucalyptus—or other natural, unheated, unrefined, organic honey, dropped by an eyedropper, or rubbed around the eye edges with the finger, to encourage penetration.

7.–According to Maryla de Chrapowicki, magnesium is useful for eye troubles. She says, "I have found magnesium helpful in many eye troubles and incipient cataracts. Ordinary Epsom salts (*mag. sulph.*) make an excellent eyewash." *Biotanic Therapy*, C. W. Daniel Co., Ashingdon, Rochford, Essex, England.)

8.–In an article in *Let's Live*[25] John Clarence Bohlender, a top-notch artist and respected officer of the Creative Arts and Crafts Guild, tells how he had been commissioned to paint a portrait of a governor, but suddenly found that he would have to give up his art since he was told by a specialist that he was developing cataracts. He moved to a farm where he could distinguish only light and dark. He also had a horse, named Old Fritz, who was going blind and the veterinarian said nothing could be done.

One day, on a psychic hunch, writes Mr. Bohlender, he felt that he should try some wild bee honey in his horse's eyes. He applied it to where he thought the horse's eyes were, since because of his own poor sight he could not see clearly, and the horse pulled, jerked and kicked when the honey entered its eyes. A few days later a neighbor examined the horse and said, "Why that old nag is all right. He can see as well as any horse."

Mr. Bohlender decided that what was good for a horse just might be good for a man, so he tried the honey on himself, which burned and stung like a thousand needles (no wonder the horse had objected). But after a few applications, the pain ceased and was replaced by a soothing, oily sensation. After about two months of three applications of honey per week, Bohlender began to see better. Improvement became more rapid; later he was able to read, and finally at eighty-five he gave up his glasses. His wife, a medical doctor, had scoffed at the honey treatment. But when she, too, developed cataracts and refused to submit to surgery, the honey treatment reversed her cataracts and she, also, was able to discard her glasses. Both of the Bohlenders now believe that a poor diet was the cause of their cataracts. When they added vitamin/mineral supplements, changed to natural foods and gave up processed products, their overall health improved.

Homeopathic Remedies

The homeopathic cell salts are an easily assimilated form of minerals. They are in tiny, sweet, white pellets which are not washed down with water, but dissolved dry on the tongue, according to dosages that appear on the label. They usually correct a mineral deficiency, and because they are rebuilt into the tissues, they take time. They are *safe* and available from some health stores and all homeopathic pharmacies.[26]

One of the cell salts recommended for cataracts by J. H. Oliver, of England, is Silicea.[27] Usually this cell salt comes in a 6x potency, but for cataracts, Dr. Oliver's suggestion is the 12x potency. This number represents the rate of trituration. *Taking twice the amount of Silicea 6x is not the same, nor will it bring the same results.* It can be ordered from the homeopathic pharmacy in the 12x potency.[28]

Calc. Fluor. (Calcium Fluoride, which is *not* the same substance as sodium fluoride added to so many state or city water supplies) has also been reported helpful, not only for cataracts but for blurred vision.[28]

A homeopathic tincture, *Cineraria Maritima,* made from an herb, has been used for years by homeopathic physicians and some ophthalmologists. One or two drops in the eye, morning and night, at the sign of any trouble, has halted and cleared some cataracts. A study by ophthalmologists shows that even in advanced cases of cataracts which had been present for four years, 22.5% of forty patients achieved good results. *Cineraria Maritima* is available only by prescription from a physician.[29]

Nutrition for Cataracts

A growing number of investigators are becoming convinced that there is a relationship between improper nutrition and cataract development.

Morgan B. Raiford, M.D., of the Atlanta, Georgia, eye clinic believes correct nutrition can help prevent cataracts. As stated earlier, he cites the cases of "sugar cataracts" in India, due to a high-carbohydrate, low-protein diet.

British scientists reported that Vitamin C is found concentrated in the lens as well as in the aqueous humor of the eye,[30] therefore a deficiency may be a factor in cataracts as well as glaucoma and other eye disturbances.

Carlton Fredericks has reported that one physician, cited in the *New England Journal of Medicine*, fed one of his patients 4,000 mgs. of Vitamin C daily for thirteen years. As a result, the patient's opacities in each eye cleared and vision was restored to 20/40 and 20/20.

The late Dr. Royal Lee said, "By proper nutritional treatment many cataracts can be removed, including traumatic cataracts. Unfortunately the time needed may extend from six months to three years. In every case the benefits obtained in general health are worth the time, independent of the effect on the cataract.

"Many patients have lost cataracts while on essential food therapy for some other ailment, indicating deficiencies were corrected. There is also evidence that cataracts, like arthritis, may be a 'cooked food disease'."

Adelle Davis has pointed out that animals develop cataracts if deprived of pantothenic acid (a B vitamin), tryptophane (an amino acid) and Vitamin B-6 needed for tryptophane assimilation. She states that our diet should be high in B-2, B-6 (plus the whole B complex as found in brewer's yeast or liver or both), pantothenic acid, Vitamins C, D, E and other nutrients.[6]

Vitamin B-2, already discussed, and given in doses of 15 mg. daily for nine months, has reversed cataracts, possibly for those with milk intolerance, and intolerance of lactose (milk sugar) or galactose.

Whey (powdered, derived from milk) has also been found to promote metabolism of galactose and lactose and inhibit cataracts in rats, according to a recent Japanese study.[31]

One testimonial came from a woman whose grandmother, at age ninety, was going blind. She was given B-2, bone meal, Vitamins A, D, C, E, protein and sunflower seed meal. At ninety-four her cataracts had disappeared and her mental and physical health were tremendously improved.

A prominent professional man had cataracts to the extent that he found it necessary to hold a page of print as close to his eyes as possible, and then read through a magnifying glass. He finally decided to go to a distant state to a clinic which specializes in cataract problems, including surgery. Although the man was prepared to have surgery, the clinic suggested that because a nutritional product—a combination of chelated magnesium and orotic acid (a rediscovered B vitamin)—had helped so many other patients, it might help him. It did. With a few short weeks on these tablets, two, three times daily, the cataractous condition had receded to the point where the man was sent home without surgery, and could read at a normal distance without the magnifying glass.[32] Meanwhile he also had improved his diet and given up milk products.

One of the most heartwarming success stories I have heard is that of an elderly aunt of a friend of mine. Aunt Laurie, a resident of a tiny, remote town in Texas, was, at age seventy-nine, diagnosed as having shaking palsy and cataracts, which, according to her doctor would require surgery. My friend lent her an electrically lighted magnifying glass to help her read, as well as some books on nutrition.

Aunt Laurie read an article which stated that adding calcium and protein to the diet had arrested some cases of cataracts. So she planned her own program, incorporated more calcium and protein into her diet. Because she had no means of transportation except once a month by relatives who lived elsewhere, she shopped only once a month. Her foods were restricted to the small town in which she lived, and because there was no health store, she ordered such provisions by mail. In spite of these problems, she religiously followed the program for five years:

1.–Two quarts of milk daily (delivered to her home).

2.–Homemade yogurt between meals.

3.–For breakfast: eggs, and a bowl of wheat germ sprinkled with brewer's yeast, anointed with corn oil, and topped with milk.

4.–Except for citrus fruits, which keep, she had almost no raw foods. She used canned turnip greens (highly nutritious) for minerals.

5.–She ate some meat, mostly canned, lots of canned tuna fish, the only fish she could get. (This was before the big mercury-contaminated tuna fish scare). She also used whole grains in some form every day.

6.–She ate every three hours, and used vitamin supplements.

7.–She took Jack La Lanne's exercises daily. At first she had to lie on the bed, because of weakness. Later she exercised sitting on the side of the bed, and still later by standing and holding on to the end of the bed. Finally she did these exercises with gusto and promptly put her relatives and friends who came to call through their paces, too, leaving them exhausted while she took the exercises in her stride.

Aunt Laurie died at ninety-four of natural causes. In spite of the fact that in the case of cataracts many are warned to avoid milk products and urged to eat a completely raw diet, she did neither. She had incredible vitality, mental alertness and had returned the loan of the lighted magnifier. She no longer had cataracts or shaking palsy (as confirmed by her doctor), and no longer needed glasses of any kind for the last ten years of her life.

This is not to say that all people should avoid milk products, or eat a raw diet; it merely means we should not generalize. Each person is different. Nutrition plus exercise solved her problem. As Aunt Laurie said, "After making a living laboratory of myself, never again will I eat for taste only."

Another case involved an elderly couple, both of whom had been diagnosed by two doctors as having cataracts which would require surgery within a year. The man and wife immediately changed their diet to include organically raised vegetables, which they grew themselves, ate fewer carbohydrates, more protein, plus lecithin, yogurt, B vitamins, especially B-2, also Vitamin A, pantothenic acid, calcium and Vitamin E supplements.

On returning to the doctor at the end of the year, he found their eyes improved and reduced the strength of their glasses. The following spring the doctor could not believe the results. In the woman, one cataract was entirely gone, the other greatly improved. The man, who had started the high nutritional diet plus supplements a little later than his wife, also showed incredible improvement. The doctor told them both they could forget about surgery, and not to come back for two years.

They did return in two years for a checkup. The doctor's verdict: "You don't need me any longer unless you have some other problem."[33]

REFERENCES
(See *Bibliography* for fuller details.)

1. John H. Tobe, *Cataract, Glaucoma and Other Eye Disorders.*
2. Linda Clark, *Are You Radioactive? How to Protect Yourself.*
3. R. Brooks Simpkins, *Science and Our Eyes.*
4. *Journal of Investigative Ophthalmology,* Vol. 5, p.65, 1966.
5. Jack Anderson's Syndicated Newspaper Column, Aug. 22, 1973.
6. Adelle Davis, *Let's Get Well.*
7. Donald T. Atkinson, M.D., "Malnutrition as an Etiological Factor in Senile Cataract." *Eye, Ear, Nose and Throat Monthly,* February, 1952.

8. *Prevention*, November, 1970.
9. *Archives of Ophthalmology*, 65, 181, 1961.
10. J.I. Rodale and Staff, *The Complete Book of Vitamins.*
11. Personal communication.
12. *Proceedings of the Society for Experimental Biology and Medicine*, Vol. 175, p. 377, 1970.
13. Irwin Stone, *The Healing Factor.*
14. Don C. Matchan, "Reflexology, 'It Works,' " *Let's Live*, November, 1973.
15. Clara A. Hackett and Lawrence Galton, *Relax and See.*
16. For information write: Cayce Membership Service, A.R.E., Box 595, Virginia Beach, Va. 23451
17. Jess Stearn, *Edgar Cayce, The Sleeping Prophet.*
18. John N. Ott, *Health and Light.*
19. R. Brooks Simpkins, *Visible Ray Therapy of the Eyes.*
20. Address: R. Brooks Simpkins, Flat 2, 7 Hardwick Road, Eastbourne, Sussex, England.
21. Linda Clark, *Know Your Nutrition.*
22. Charles Perry, *New Beauty.*
23. M. O. Garten, N.D., *The Health Secrets of a Naturopathic Doctor.*
24. Claudia V. James, *That Old Green Magic.*
25. John Clarence Bohlender, "Eyesight Restored Through Honey and a Blind Horse," *Let's Live*, September, 1965.
26. If no homeopathic pharmacy is in your area, write for information to Standard Homeopathic Pharmacy, P.O. Box 61067, Los Angeles, Cal., 90061.
27. J. H. Oliver, *Proven Remedies.*
28. Inez Eudora Perry and George Washington Carey, *The Zodiac and the Salts of Salvation.*
29. Richard Lucas, *The Magic of Herbs in Daily Living.*
30. *British Journal of Nutrition*, November, 1971.
31. Japanese Journal of Pharmacology, 1, 21, 97–106, 1971.
32. For information write: Millar Pharmacal, Box 299, West Chicago, Ill. 60185.
33. "Avoiding Cataract Surgery." *Let's Live*, August, 1971.

10: GLAUCOMA

(And Other Eye Problems)

Glaucoma is a disease of the eye characterized by an increase of pressure within the eyeball (called intraocular pressure). It is similar to, though has no connection with, high blood pressure in the body. A certain amount of intraocular pressure is considered acceptable, but too much is associated with damage to the eye, and vision loss may occur. Detection by an eye doctor at regular intervals is important since glaucoma can sneak up without warning, and measures to prevent further vision loss are vitally important since eye experts believe that such vision loss cannot be repaired.[1]

I always hesitate to give symptoms of any ailment since one can imagine himself, through the subconscious, into almost any disease.[2] However, the usual symptoms of glaucoma (among others) include seeing colored halos around lights, a loss of peripheral or side vision, intermittent headaches and eyeaches, dim or fuzzy vision which comes and goes, particularly after excess exposure in long hours of darkness to television and

119

movies.[1] Many eye researchers also believe glaucoma to be psychosomatic (caused by the mind).[3,4]

The cause of glaucoma apparently varies. It can be hereditary since it has been found to run in families. But for unknown reasons it can also result from a blockage of the drainage canal, causing the aqueous humor (eye fluid) to back up and create the build-up of pressure within the eye.[1] Farsighted people appear to be more prone to glaucoma than nearsighted ones.[3]

Glaucoma has also been blamed on defective circulation of nutrients to the eye, and associated with giddiness, sinus conditions, allergies, diabetes, hypoglycemia, arteriosclerosis (cholesterol deposits) and an imbalance of the autonomic nervous system as well as disturbed pituitary function. It has sometimes followed the use of antispasmodic or steroid (cortisone) drugs. Emotional stress has been found to be a definite predisposing factor in glaucoma. General body health is basic to all of these conditions.

Therapy is initiated to preserve what slight remains and fortunately there are hopeful and helpful measures to use.

Orthodox doctors employ eye drops for local control of the eye, and, if that fails, oral drugs.

There are some substances which almost all eye specialists agree are no-nos for glaucoma patients. One of these is coffee. Most specialists absolutely forbid the use of coffee because of its caffeine content. (Decaffeinated coffee is allowed.) Beer and tobacco, which can cause blood vessel constriction, are also forbidden.[3,4] The amount of liquid allowed is restricted by many doctors.[1]

Certain nutritional substances have been found helpful. Glaucoma patients are usually deficient in Vitamins A, B, C, protein, calcium and other minerals. Since highstrung individuals are more apt to be candidates for glaucoma, nutrients such as calcium and B complex, which relieve stress, appear also to relieve the intraocular condition. Additional rest periods, vacations, and relaxation on a regular basis are also advisable. Adelle Davis stated that every case of glaucoma with which she worked was cleared up. Her program included her antistress formula (given on p. 26 of her book *Let's Get Well*) six times daily, plus Vitamin B-2 (riboflavin), and, surprisingly, in addition to an adequate diet, salt or salty foods. (Whole, natural sea salt may be safer than the usual sodium chloride found in most salt shakers.)[5] She told of the case of one man whose glaucoma in both eyes quickly disappeared and had not returned after increasing his intake of salt. This man had previously been forbidden salt because of a heart condition, yet one physician prescribes whole sea salt, added to water, to be sipped daily to revive hearts and prevent attacks!

Adelle Davis did warn that if an adequate diet is not continued, the glaucoma may return. Ethel Maslansky, a former nutritionist of the New York City Department of Health, found that the use of protein, Vitamin A and niacin should always be ample in the diet.[5] One of the most dramatic treatments of glaucoma is Vitamin C. At a meeting of the Roman Opthalmological Society in Rome, Italy, research was reported by doctors showing that the intraocular pressure in glaucoma could be lowered amazingly, regardless of the cause or type of glaucoma, by Vitamin C therapy. Dr. Michele Virno and his coworkers reported that the average person weighing 150 pounds, given seven thousand mg. of ascorbic acid, five times daily (or 35,000 mg. in all, per day), acquired acceptable intraocular pressure within forty-five days. Symptoms such as mild stomach discomfort and diarrhea from the large doses of C were temporary and soon disappeared.[1]

Fred R. Klenner, M.D., who has done years of research with Vitamin C therapy recommends that some calcium should always be taken with each dose of ascorbic acid used for any purpose to minimize or prevent any possible side effects of the large doses.

Professor G. B. Bietti, director of the Eye Clinic of the University of Rome, confirmed the following findings of the Vitamin C therapy for glaucoma: Vitamin C was found not only helpful, but safe in the large doses recommended for glaucoma; it is inexpensive; it is safer than eye drops or oral drugs; and it may preserve sight after all drugs and surgery have failed.[1]

Another study using rutin, usually found in the bioflavonoids, or whole Vitamin C complex (of which ascorbic acid is but one factor) was successful on most of the twenty-six patients treated to whom a 20-milligram dose of rutin was given three times daily. The pressure in seventeen of the subjects was reduced, whereas four were not aware whether or not a change had occurred, and five did not notice any results. The length of time of the study was eight months.[6]

In their book, *New Hope for Incurable Diseases*, E. Cheraskin, M.D., and W. M. Ringsdorf, Jr. give a list of suggestions for glaucoma patients. Here it is in partial form only, due to lack of space. (The complete list is truly beneficial).[1]

1.–Avoid excessive use of stimulants such as coffee and tea. Drink no more than ½ to 1 cup of coffee daily. You may drink caffeine-free coffee.

2.–Avoid excessive liquid at any one time. Even in hot weather, if you are thirsty, do not drink three or four glasses at once; spread them out.

3.–Avoid excessive smoking.

4.–Lead as tranquil a life as possible.

5.–Avoid prolonged periods of darkness (T.V., movies, etc.) and do not overdo the use of dark glasses outdoors.

6.–Ordinary use of eyes for reading, sewing, and television watching does not damage your eyes.

7.–Watch out for allergies, particularly to drugs.

There is still further help available from unexpected quarters, perhaps as yet undiscovered by many orthodox practitioners. Please reread the portion on color therapy for the eyes in the cataract chapter in which Mr. Simpkins of England states that exposure to the correct shade of green color has been helpful for glaucoma. He says, "The raised intraocular pressure usually goes down within ten minutes after exposure (to the green light treatments)."[7] Unfortunately, color therapy is not allowed in the

United States, not because it is not safe, but because orthodoxy refuses to believe that it can be helpful.[8]

The Bates system of eye exercise has helped many, although eye experts sometimes scoff at eye exercises. However, I know of several doctors who recommend them for their patients, with excellent results. The most helpful do-it-yourself book on these exercises I have found is called *Relax and See*, by Clara A. Hackett and Lawrence Galton, published by Faber and Faber in London, England but now available in the U.S. through your own bookstore.[10]

The book gives exercises for increasing your peripheral, or side vision, soon lost in glaucoma. It also outlines a step-by-step 12-week program of exercises for the relief of glaucoma itself. There are three pages of case histories of people who have received vision improvement, as well as lowered intraocular pressure, all confirmed by their eye specialists, by this system.

Clara Hackett also suggests a light treatment for glaucoma. She says to let the sun shine through your closed eyelids for two minutes at a time, as you turn your head slowly from side to side. A doctor with early glaucoma reversed his condition in himself by this method, she reports.

The price of the book is moderate and a small amount of pay for improved vision and glaucoma control, or any eye problem, in fact.

Other Eye Problems

This same book, mentioned above, also gives information on rehabilitating the eyes for general vision improvement. The author explains how to improve ocular fusion, how to learn to see clearly at all distances, as well as in reading. She gives step-by-step programs for nearsightedness, farsightedness, crossed eyes, color blindness, bifocal wearers and other eye problems, both simple and serious.

Nutrition has come to the rescue in many eye ailments. Adelle Davis wrote, "Blurred vision, produced in volunteers deficient in

Vitamins B-6 and pantothenic acid, was quickly corrected when these vitamins were given."[5] She added that weak eye muscles, crossed eyes, blurred or double vision have responded to Vitamin E, or liver, or brewer's yeast, and that retinitis has been corrected by a high protein diet.

Vitamin A has been found internationally to improve night vision. Pilots and military personnel are now required, in some cases, to take it daily. It is said that the French feed their pilots blueberries.

The bioflavonoids (Vitamin C complex) have been used with great success for eye hemorrhages, as well as for blood oozing from broken capillaries or the retina in diabetic patients. Such cases have responded favorably, as reported by Catharyn Elwood in her book, *Feel Like a Million*.[11] The chapter on Vitamin P (another name for the bioflavonoids) and its many successful results is an exciting one.

I received a letter recently from a man who had suffered from glaucoma for many years. And he admitted that he had "tried everything" with no success until he discovered using natural, filtered, sea water in his eyes as eye drops. (This is available from health stores and is taken from deep sea depths to avoid contamination.)

The letter read, "Just a brief note to tell you I had a glaucoma check yesterday, the first in two years. The pressure in both eyes was 18, which, as the doctor said, is perfect.

When the doctor asked me what I had been doing, I told him I had been using sea water drops in my eyes, morning and night. He said if I thought it was helping, to continue its use as long as it was purified (meaning filtered)."

The Schuessler cell salt, *Calc. Fluor*, has been used for blurred vision, and *Nat. Phos.* for vision which fluctuates from day to day, "cloudy today, clearer tomorrow," according to Inez Eudora Perry.[12] Since all of the twelve cell salts are easily assimilated forms of minerals, I would not be without a single one of them.

They are available from all homeopathic pharmacies and some health stores.

One homeopathic physician has been extremely successful in reversing glaucoma. This physician has found that glaucoma can result from a malfunctioning hypothalamus gland and supplies the homeopathic substance *gelsemium* with success.

No discussion of eyes and vision would be complete without the mention of the work of Dr. John Nash Ott. He has spent over forty years in researching the effect of light on plants, animals, people, and especially eyes in response to light. He states that we are behind glass so much of the time—windows, windshields, eyeglases—that the natural sunlight, which is partially filtered out by ordinary glass, cannot reach our eyes. He reports the case of a photographer who nearly became blind from spending so many hours in the darkroom, and had some sight restored after gradually becoming accustomed to more hours in the sunlight. Dr. Ott's own case of arthritis cleared after he broke his sunglasses, which he frowns upon for health of the body as well as the eyes. Light that enters the eyes can help both body and vision, he says. You will find the full story in my book on color therapy,[8] or in John Ott's own book, *Health and Light.*[9]

Sometimes eyesight is affected by neck tension, which can be relieved by stretching the neck and turning it widely first three times in a clockwise direction, followed by three times in a counterclockwise direction. Jess Stearn, in his book on Edgar Cayce,[13] tells of definite eye improvement in many people who do this exercise *every day*, at least for six months. A chiropractor or osteopath can also relieve the atlas or axis at the base of the back of the neck should they be out of alignment. Eyes are easily affected by constriction in this area, and often relieved by proper alignment, a fact to which many people can testify.

Eyes are among our most precious possessions. Feed them, exercise them, relax them, and respect them. In return, they will pay you many dividends.

REFERENCES
(See *Bibliography* for fuller details.)

1. E. Cheraskin, M.D., D.M.D., and Wm. Ringsdorf, Jr., D.M.D., M.S., *New Hope for Incurable Diseases*.
2. Linda Clark, *Help Yourself to Health*.
3. John H. Tobe, *Cataract, Glaucoma and Other Eye Disorders*.
4. J. I. Rodale and Staff, *Encyclopedia of Common Diseases*.
5. Adelle Davis, *Let's Get Well*.
6. Bicknell and Prescott, *The Vitamins in Medicine*.
7. R. Brooks Simpkins, *Visible Ray Therapy of the Eyes*.
8. Linda Clark, *Color Therapy*.
9. John N. Ott, *Health and Light*.
10. Clara A. Hackett and Lawrence Galton, *Relax and See*.
11. Catharyn Elwood, *Feel Like a Million*.
12. Inez Eudora Perry and George Washington Carey, *The Zodiac and the Salts of Salvation*.
13. Jess Stearn, *Edgar Cayce, The Sleeping Prophet*.

11: CONSTIPATION

Constipation is a big bore. But people who complain about it are bigger bores, particularly when constipation is so easy to correct!

Constipation is a favorite mental preoccupation or topic of conversation amongst the elderly in retirement centers where people congregate in the common rooms, on the patios or even on park benches and will worry aloud to anyone who will listen to their hopes for a bowel movement that day. The only listeners who are not bored are the delighted laxative manufacturers who promise, via their commercials, to "keep you regular."

Buncombe! Laxatives and cathartics can *cause* constipation, creating a vicious cycle by causing a dependence on still more laxatives, and a gradual weakening of the body's own nerves and muscular control which are constructed to do the work if given a fair chance. Also, laxatives not only irritate intestinal membranes, but interfere with digestion and assimilation by rushing the food through in such a hurry that the body cannot benefit from it. Fortunately the message has finally got through to the public and the medical profession that mineral oil is one of the most damaging of all laxatives. It robs the body of Vitamins A, D, E, K; interferes with the absorption of calcium and phosphorus, and can actually lead to other diseases. Another dangerous laxative, according to the late Dr. Royal Lee, is milk of magnesia, which can cause nose bleeds.[1]

As Catharyn Elwood says, "Enemas, high colonics and some of the milder herbal laxatives are recommended—but only when absolutely necessary."[2] *Any* regular, artificial eliminative means merely weakens the body's own control. Miss Elwood adds, "Remember, *your nerves move your bowels.*" This shows that constipation can be not only a physical problem, but a psychological one. Worry itself can paralyze intestinal traffic by tensing those controlling nerves.

What is the solution to the problem? The concept is really quite simple. Anthropologists who have studied various worldwide tribes from earliest history down to the present time, have learned that those (animals *and* people) who stay close to nature are the most free of disease. Conversely, we find today that those who live on refined "civilized foods" are the most prone to disease. This is not armchair gossip. For example, Stefansson found that the Eskimos who lived on fish and other native foods had no tooth decay. Later, when the trading posts were opened by the white man, and white flour and white sugar became available, cavities appeared in the Eskimos for the first time in history. Even those healthy Hunzas who are now yielding to the temptations of imported refined foods are paying for it with poorer health, according to reports from some recent visitors to Hunzaland. Refined foods can cause constipation, as you will see.

Do you realize how many ailments have already responded to natural food substances? Scurvy, a Vitamin C-deficiency disease, yielded to citrus fruits, not to a drug.

Beri-beri, which caused blind staggers in prisoners and chickens after eating white rice, was relieved not by a drug, but by whole brown rice or the Vitamin B-rich rice polishings that had been removed, leaving the rice white and denuded of Vitamin B.

Pellagra, which formerly caused 10,000 deaths annually in the southern United States, yielded not to a drug, but to niacin, a B vitamin which had been removed from cornmeal by food refiners.

Many cases of coronary thrombosis (causing heart attacks), according to Wilfrid E. Shute, M.D., have been traced to the millers' removal of wheat germ, containing the protective Vitamin E.

And rickets have been controlled not by drugs, but by Vitamins A and D found in cod liver and other fish oils.[3]

Those of the opposition who defend refined or synthetic foods and call us who are interested in nutrition "food faddists," apparently forget these examples, medically documented. They also make fun of us for taking the supplements they have removed from the food, and condemn us for trying to get natural, organic food, which is uncontaminated by the insecticides and other poisons they have tried to sell us.

What does all of this have to do with constipation? Everything! Fresh, whole, natural food, and its components, are the keystone to correcting constipation which was probably caused by its lack in the first place. So listen closely to these simple corrective measures:

Constipation can be prevented, or has been corrected, by a natural diet used for a least a thousand years. It consists of unrefined foods such as:

—Fruits and vegetables, preferably fresh and raw to supply bulk as well as the mineral, potassium, and prevent a hard stool.

—Plenty of protein such as meats, eggs, cheese, and nuts, to strengthen intestinal muscles.

—Whole grains, rich in B vitamins which are needed by nerves to control elimination naturally.

—Soured milks to help the body manufacture more B vitamins in the intestines as well as to help establish a healthy intestinal flora which can correct constipation.

If these all-natural food sources of a vitamin/mineral supply are missing in the diet, then individual vitamins and minerals are needed:

1.–Pantothenic acid, (B-5) as well as all other B vitamins.[4]

2.–The mineral potassium, the lack of which can slow down intestinal muscle contractions partially or completely. Adelle Davis writes, "Potassium is essential to the contraction of every muscle in the body . . . weak muscles of the intestines allow bacteria to form quantities of gas."[4]

Sugar and sugary foods should be strictly avoided because sugar steals B vitamins from the body, and without B vitamins, the intestines cannot function normally.

One food which is an excellent source of B vitamins, minerals (including potassium) *and* protein is brewer's yeast. Some people find their constipation problem solved by the use of this one food alone, taken daily in juice or water or in a health drink. But there are some tips to observe here. Occasionally when a person first tries brewer's yeast, he may develop large amounts of gas. There is more than one reason for this. If the intestinal flora are invaded by unfriendly bacteria, and a source friendly to flora (such as brewer's yeast) is introduced, war results. There is a battle royal between the two floras—good and bad—until one of them over-populates the other and wins the war.

Gas results from this battle.

One method to stop and win the war is not to give up but to continue taking the brewer's yeast plus other sources of the friendly bacteria to help vanquish the unfriendly bacteria. Faster help comes from soured milks such as cultured buttermilk and yogurt. If results are really serious, then acidophilus culture in liquid form taken between or with each meal will do the job quickly. Acidophilus contains millions of live, friendly organisms in liquid form, and helps quickly to re-establish the normal intestinal flora. (It is available from health stores.)

Antibiotics kill the friendly intestinal flora. Italian and other European doctors understand this and if they feel an antibiotic is necessary, they prescribe simultaneously with the antibiotic, yogurt, or acidophilus to protect the patient's healthy intestinal flora.

Another cause of gas is undigested protein. Protein requires acid for digestion. Hydrochloric acid taken after a protein meal, or with brewer's yeast which is high in protein, usually eliminates the gas resulting from such indigestion. The correct dosage and type of HCL, as explained by a doctor, are discussed in my book, *Secrets of Health and Beauty* (in paperback at health and book stores). If you are unable to procure the HCL, apple cider vinegar, diluted with water and taken with each meal can suffice, at least temporarily.

Other digestive enzymes may be necessary. If the diet is low in protein, high in *refined* (man-made) carbohydrates, little bile can be manufactured. Even if bile flow is restricted by a congestion in the gall bladder, a hard stool can result. Many people favor a low-fat diet, yet little or no fat can be *dangerous* and actually cause gallstones, since the gall bladder *must have some fat to stimulate its activity and manufacture bile*. Adelle Davis adds, "In addition to taking some fat, digestive enzymes with bile and hydrochloric acid should be used to insure greater protein absorption and the soured milks or acidophilus taken to destroy gas forming intestinal bacteria."[4]

Intestinal bacteria, and resulting gas, also multiply tremendously on undigested foods. Not only are the digestive aids indicated here important, but a rediscovery of an anticonstipation substance has recently attracted the attention of doctors and laymen alike. Again we return to a natural food which this time is conquering many intestinal problems. Diseases such as diverticulitis including tremendous amounts of gas; gall stones; irritable colons; even intestinal cancer have been found to result from too little fiber in the diet, and to respond to an old friend discovered years ago and removed from whole grains, *bran*.

Dr. Neil Painter, surgeon of Manor House Hospital, London, states, "Bran can save a lot of dangerous surgical operations. Bran is both safe and cheap."

Dr. Kenneth Heaton, a consulting physician at Bristol University, England, states that bran can sweep the intestines clean of gall bladder by-products, remove undigested food (as in diverticulitis) and relieve other disturbing conditions resulting from a bland and refined carbohydrate diet. Bran can bring relief to the vast majority of patients, he believes.

Dr. Dennis Burkitt, a British surgeon from South Africa, reports that white races with their low-fiber diet derived from "civilized, refined foods" have some of the highest incidence of intestinal diseases in the world, compared with nonexistence of these intestinal diseases among the black population who live on a high fiber diet and suffer little from constipation.

A study was conducted in England by Dr. Neil Painter and associates using a diet of generous amounts of natural food fiber in the form of fruits, vegetables, coarse whole grain bread, *plus bran.* In addition, the patients were warned to reduce their intake of sugar in any form. The results of the study are near-sensational as reported in the *British Medical Journal,* April 15, 1972:

The following ailments were abolished in the majority of patients given the high fiber diet:
—Constipation
—Tender rectum
—Highly odorous gas
—Heartburn, nausea and bloating

Dr. Burkitt also reports a lowered cholesterol and fewer cases of coronary thrombosis from the addition of bran.

Dr. Burkitt believes that today's typical diet of highly refined, low-fiber foods leads to slow-moving bowels and small, hard feces. He has found with numerous patients that a diet high in unrefined foods and fiber leads to faster bowel transit time and large, soft feces.

Even doctors are now taking bran! The doctor-recommended use of unprocessed, natural 100% bran (removed during milling from wheat or rice) apparently owes its success, in part, to the fact that bran absorbs large amounts of water and produces larger and softer stools. Catharyn Elwood has recommended for a dry stool an intake of eight to ten glasses of liquids in the form of water, juices, or natural beverages every day.[2] This need for liquid may become still more important if bran is added, due to its uptake of water.

How much bran should you take? Dr. Painter suggests that one should begin with a small amount at first. Sprinkle it on cereal or salads, or put in juices or a protein drink. If you add it to baked goods such as bread and muffins, this is fine, except that it is hard to know how much each person in the family gets, particularly when different people may need different amounts.

The type of bran used is in small flake form, not the rough type as of yore. The flaked bran (usually at health stores) is gentle and does not irritate the colon.

Meanwhile, I utilize bran in muffins which I make for breakfast as follows:

1 cup unbleached flour
1 cup bran flakes
3 teaspoons of baking powder
1 cup milk
1 egg
3 tablespoons of oil
Approximately ¼ cup honey

Combine the dry ingredients. Blend all liquids with egg in blender and stir into dry ingredients. You may add blueberries (fresh or frozen), nuts, sunflower seeds, raisins, or whatever, to vary the flavor.

Bake at 400° for 20 minutes.

This recipe makes twelve muffins. If you live alone, left over muffins can be individually dampened and warmed in the oven. If your family is larger, there will not be any left over. They are delicious.

Dr. Painter suggests that you start with one or two teaspoons of bran a day and increase until you find the amount best for you. The best average amount was found to be about two teaspoons three times daily. When you first begin the bran, the doctors warn that you may temporarily experience some flatulence and distention, which should disappear within a few weeks, so don't give up too early. However, there may be a few people who cannot tolerate bran at all. If so, the high fiber from the fresh fruits and vegetables can be relied upon.

This natural diet, described so far, and of growing interest, is the type to eat day in and day out to prevent, as well as reverse, bowel troubles. *It should be a way of life.* Meanwhile there are some safe emergency measures to use if you need them. Blackstrap molasses, used in very small amounts (as needed by each person) is a powerful laxative. It is full of minerals, particularly potassium. It should be added to liquids, not taken by the spoon, since it clings to the teeth, possibly causing tooth decay as any concentrated sweet can do. Prunes and figs, though laxative in effect, contain concentrated sugars with the same drawback. Use them for emergencies, not as regular additions to the diet.

Another help: chew one tablespoon of whole flaxseed daily and swallow quickly with liquid before the seeds become thick. They become gelatinous and increase in bulk in the intestines. You may pulverize them in a blender or a small nut-grinding mill, but do it freshly just before use each day. Flaxseed, once broken and exposed to the air can become rancid quickly. (The whole seed does not.)

Still another excellent method of overcoming constipation is the use of clay water, taken internally, as described in that delightful book, *Our Earth, Our Cure,* published by Swan House Publishers, Box 170, Brooklyn, N.Y. 11223. If your health stores do not yet have the book, ask them to order it for you. The source of the clay is listed in the buyer's guide at the back of the book. I, and all of my friends who have tried it, can testify that it works like a charm.

If you really have a serious emergency, here is an isotonic solution: one teaspoonful of table salt added to a pint of water and drunk down quickly first thing in the morning will give you a quick flush-out within an hour, unless you are deficient in salt, in which case you may need more salt.[1] But again, do not do this often, since it washes out many beneficial nutrients if used on a regular basis.

Many people suffer from hemorrhoids as a result of a hard stool or straining. Two natural remedies for this problem are either a peeled clove of garlic, or a piece of whittled raw potato about the size of a garlic clove inserted at night into the rectum. The best remedy of all, however, is suggested by Alan H. Nittler, M.D. in his book.[5] This is Collinsonia Root Powder in capsule form, put out by Standard Process Products, a subsidiary of Vitamin Products Co., Milwaukee, Wisconsin. These products are available *only through doctors* of any kind: M.D.'s, D.C.'s, D.O.'s, N.D.'s—even dentists. I have heard people rave enthusiastically about the results of this remedy, which works quickly.

Don't forget that exercise of any type that will stimulate and strengthen abdominal muscles, is a logical help for constipation. Walking, swimming, bowling, gardening (which involves bending), golf, etc., or whatever your choice, are beneficial.

Finally, there are those who never use an alarm clock to wake themselves in the morning. They merely issue an order to their subconscious mind the night before, stating the time they wish to be awakened. You can do the same thing with scheduling a bowel movement. At night give your subconscious the directions for the desired time and type (early, complete, etc.). At first, to get the attention of your subconscious, you may have to repeat the directive three times, without any feeling of worry or concern. In time, the subconscious will get the message and should quickly respond.

Meanwhile, look for another topic of worrisome thought or conversation. If you follow the suggestions given here, you won't need this one any more.

Summary of Constipation Remedies
Brewer's yeast
Clay
Fiber, including fresh, raw fruits, vegetables and bran flakes
Adequate water
Adequate protein
Whole grains

Soured milks
B vitamins, especially pantothenic acid
Minerals, especially potassium (found in green leafy vegetables)
Blackstrap molasses
Whole flaxseed
Avoid sugar and sugar products and mineral oil
Emergency treatment: isotonic solution

REFERENCES
(See *Bibliography* for fuller details.)

1. Royal Lee, D.D.S., "The Constipation Syndrome." *Let's Live*, March, 1962.
2. Catharyn Elwood, "Overcoming Constipation." *Let's Live*, May, 1962.
3. Linda Clark, *Know Your Nutrition*.
4. Adelle Davis, *Let's Get Well*.
5. Alan H. Nittler, M.D., *A New Breed of Doctor*. Chap. 12

12: DIARRHEA

As you already know, diarrhea is the opposite of constipation. With constipation, you can't get started. With diarrhea, you can't stop.

Diarrhea is no joke, as anyone who has had it will testify. It has been grimly nicknamed by tourists—who are particularly susceptible to it, especially while traveling in foreign countries—as *Turista,* or *Montezuma's Revenge* (Mexico), *Delhi Belly* (India), and most recently by the medical name *Giardiasis* (Russia). (More about this last one later.) But diarrhea can hit you in your own country, even in your own home, which is not news to you.

When diarrhea strikes, most people are not only taken by surprise; they are not prepared to deal with it. How often have you said, "Oh, what *was* the remedy for diarrhea I heard about not long ago?" but in your understandable state of agitation, you can't remember it. So keep this chapter in mind as a handy reference for the future . . . just in case.

Sometimes you will be able to choose the right remedy on the first try, *if* you will do a little self-searching of what you have been eating, drinking, or breathing. Otherwise you may have to go down the line of remedies, one by one, by trial and error until you find it. So before you begin, it is a time-saver to know what can cause diarrhea.

Causes of Diarrhea

Diarrhea usually means that there is something taking refuge in your intestinal tract which shouldn't be there. It may be due to "something in the water"—most common in foreign countries—but with the influx of pollution in our own country, not exactly unheard of here. The peculiar thing is that in most foreign countries, the natives do not suffer like the tourists. In India, for example, the natives seem to be immune to whatever may be in the water, whereas non-native newcomers, even those who have lived in India for some time, are felled by one misstep. They can boil their drinking water, or use water purifying tablets from pharmacies, all with success. But if they become forgetful and wash their teeth with tap water even once, the curse is upon them!

Because the body may have built up its own immunity to tolerate water in its own community, this does not mean one can get away with drinking water anywhere else, even just one hundred miles distant where the condition of the water may be entirely different. This explains why so many football teams have carried their own water with them when they travel to a distant state for a game. Coaches have learned by experience that a bout of diarrhea can lose a game with no other odds against them. This knowledge also explains why Presidents and potentates travelling abroad carry their own water with them.

Other common causes of diarrhea include parasites, germs, a virus, bacteria or micro-organism of some kind, or a poison which has sneaked into the body via food, water or air, and isn't about to leave without an argument. Summertime diarrhea, resulting from gastroenteritis, is common. I have seen it develop in communities almost in epidemic form, leaving doctors helpless with no other diagnosis than "something going around." Due to my suspicious nature about chemicals, I have often wondered if the cause might be due to sprays taking a free ride into the markets on various produce. This is not as impossible as it sounds. One alert doctor once found that a "strange" virus (named virus X) affecting soldiers during the early Vietnam war was caused by spraying the environment with DDT.

Food poisoning, of course, has caused much trouble. Even underripe summer fruit picked and shipped green, as well as the well-known green, underripe apples, can cause diarrhea. I recall hearing a doctor in a small midwestern town where all fruit was shipped in, state that he made more money in the summertime from treating his patients for diarrhea resulting from eating underripe fruit, than the grower, the shipper or the retailer of the fruit.

Diarrhea can also result from an allergy. Many years ago, one woman noticed that her diarrhea was seasonal, occurring during the Christmas holidays only. She finally learned that it was due to citron in fruit cake, and after the fruit cake season was over, so was her diarrhea. Another person, learning that her diarrhea was caused by allergy to milk, has used regularly one teaspoon of milk daily as a laxative. In these days of chemicals in and on everything, you really have to be a detective. But the search may pay you valuable dividends.

Dysentery

Dysentery, although somewhat similar to diarrhea, is a different ailment. It is considered an infectious disease, often spread because of poor sanitation and perhaps characterized by ulcerative inflammation of the colon, sometimes causing bloody stools. It can be caused by a certain bacillus, or by a protozoon, as in amoebic dysentery, which is often picked up in foreign countries and may hang on for years. This is a case for the doctor since it may be serious. However, one report states that 500 mg. of Vitamin C in combination with other treatment used daily by the Russians "rapidly eliminated the clinical symptoms of severe dysentery, led to more favorable progress, and shortened the duration of the illness."[1] Irwin Stone, who reports this study comments that if as little as 500 mg. daily could produce such improvement, megavitamin doses could do still better.

Why Diarrhea Can be Serious

Those who try to look on the bright side of diarrhea and consider it a good chance to become detoxified or lose weight (which you will gain back anyway), had better pull up short and realize that there are some health dangers at work here. Why?

1.–Weakening takes place. Nutrients are lost. Blood sugar drops, producing hypoglycemia symptoms.

2.–Food is rushed through the body without giving the nutrients a chance to be absorbed. Vitamins A, D, E, and K are lost.

3.–Loss of body fluids leads to dehydration.

4.–Most important of all, minerals are washed out of the body:

—Iron loss, if the diarrhea continues, can lead to anemia.

—Too much calcium loss can lead to softer bones and teeth, irritable nerves.

—Magnesium is washed out of the body, causing nervous conditions. Magnesium supplements can help here. (See your health food store.)

—Potassium is eliminated, one of the most serious effects of all. Potassium regulates muscle contractions necessary to *stop* the onrush of the ailment. Its lack creates a condition somewhat similar to a train running downhill without any brakes. Extra potassium is called for immediately. (Ask your health store or druggist.)

—Sodium is lost. One of the first symptoms of the loss of sodium is a weary, "washed-out" feeling. According to John E. Eichenlaub, M.D., this can and should be corrected as fast as possible by taking extra salt (whole sea salt from health stores is best) added to drinking water. Eating salty foods will also help, he says.[2]

In addition to replacing lost minerals, here are some diarrhea remedies which have proved helpful:

Acid: The late D. C. Jarvis of folk medicine fame, has stated that germs or bacteria *cannot live in an acid medium.* He advised his patients to add two teaspoons of apple cider vinegar to a glassful of water whenever there was a question of safety of any food to be eaten. He tells of people who ate the same food at some church suppers and large picnics where food was prepared in advance and kept warm or unrefrigerated for unlimited time. Those whom he had taught to drink apple cider vinegar in water did not contract diarrhea. Others did. Apple cider vinegar can be used as a prevention, but Dr. Jarvis also used it as a remedy, once diarrhea had taken hold. In one case he used it successfully for another doctor who was stricken with diarrhea plus vomiting, at a medical convention. From a mixture of a glassful of water plus one teaspoonful of apple cider vinegar, he gave the man a teaspoonful every five minutes. He mixed a second glassful in the same way and gave him two teaspoons every five minutes. The third glassful he told the doctor to take one small swallow every fifteen minutes. The doctor recovered and ate his supper. In fact, Dr. Jarvis said that if you would follow this routine if you awaken with diarrhea and vomiting in the morning, you, too, will be ready to eat a small meal of easily digested food by evening. He recommends continuing the vinegar-in-water with meals for two or three days afterward.[3]

The reason Dr. Jarvis gave the apple cider vinegar and water in small doses for this ailment is because he found the stomach would not accept a whole glassful at one time, whereas a teaspoonful or more could be kept down (in case of vomiting).

Dr. E. Hugh Tuckey used a different type of acid to prevent and control "turista" for those who traveled to Mexico. He advocated hydrochloric acid. (The type and the dosage are explained in my book, *Secrets of Health and Beauty.*[4] Lack of space prevents repeating it here.)

European folk medicine prescribes lemon juice, taken straight (but wash your teeth afterward to prevent enamel erosion); or strong black coffee.

Herbs: Herbal remedies for diarrhea abound, as you will see if you pick up any herb book. One, cayenne pepper, also known as capsicum, can be sprinkled on juice or food or put into an empty capsule. It also acts as a vermifuge if parasites or worms have caused the diarrhea. Cayenne belongs to the paprika family and is rich in Vitamin P, another name for the whole Vitamin C complex, or bioflavonoids. But it has additional values.

Camomile tea has arrested diarrhea in calves.[5]

As stomach soothers, as well as to help allay the diarrhea itself, comfrey (which is mucilagenous), slippery elm tea, and arrowroot dissolved in water have been used. Honey is soothing as well as a germ killer, providing it is unrefined.

One product found invaluable because it *ad*sorbs (draws out) toxins and poisons from the intestines, is a clay gel. I know a doctor who travels and lectures extensively. He feels it is not safe to travel without this type of product these days.[6]

The use of clay water, taken internally, explained in the previous chapter on constipation, has been found to eliminate parasites, amoebic dysentery, as well as diarrhea. It is a simple, yet powerful remedy. It also adsorbs and eliminates toxins, parasites and poisons from the body.

John E. Eichenlaub, M.D. recommends the well-known products from the pharmacies which contain kaolin and pectin. He warns not to buy those compounded with antispasmodics, which he considers dangerous.[2]

Other remedies which have been proved effective by doctors are carrot soup, bananas, turmeric powder, carob, and certain vitamin supplements.[7]

Carrot soup was used by a Swedish doctor, P. Selander, M.D., who also reported excellent results from Germany, France and Belgium. An American doctor, Carl L. Thenebe, M.D., treated diarrhea and enteritis in hospitals and homes of 600 sufferers with good results in every case.[8] He also used it successfully with acute colitis. The explanation for the success of the carrot soup makes sense: it supplies water to combat dehydration, replenishes sodium, potassium, phosphorus, calcium, sulphur, magnesium, supplies pectin and coats the intestines to allay inflammation. It checks the growth of harmful intestinal bacteria and prevents vomiting. It is especially good for children. Here is the recipe:

One pound of carrots cooked in five ounces or more water until soft. Strain the pulp or blend in a blender and add boiled water to make a quart. Add ¾ tablespoon salt (very important for providing sodium). Give small amounts every half hour. Improvement is usually noticed in 24 hours.

Bananas have replaced the old home remedy of scraped apple. Studies have shown that children treated with mashed bananas recovered faster than controls who did not take bananas. The explanation is that bananas contain pectin and encourage the growth of beneficial bacteria.[9] Recently, however, many find themselves becoming allergic to bananas. This problem is explained later, with a solution.

The use of carob flour for diarrhea in both children and adults has been hailed as one of the greatest antidiarrheal steps in recent years. Studies show that one to five doses of carob flour added to hot water (it tastes like chocolate) controlled 60% of infectious diarrhea and 95% of noninfectious diarrhea. Recovery time was definitely shortened.[10]

Turmeric, a yellow vegetable powder used as a condiment in India, was tested in one study of thirty patients with diarrhea. Diarrhea was checked in twenty-two of the patients within seventy-two hours.[11]

Boiled milk has long been a standby for diarrhetic babies, but Boston's Childrens' Hospital now frowns on the practice,[12] whereas doctors at Duke University Medical School highly recommend acidified milk such as yogurt, or lactic acid buttermilk for controlling diarrhea and dysentery for both adults and children.[13]

This is probably the greatest remedy of all for several reasons. The soured or cultured milks help overcome disturbing intestinal flora, and re-establish the benign or friendly flora, which in turn helps the intestines to help themselves. The acid in the soured milks also fights germs and bacteria. If taking small amounts of yogurt or lactic acid buttermilk does not bring desired results fast enough, a stronger, but safe product can speed the results: acidophilus, found in liquid form at health stores. It contains millions of live friendly bacteria which go to work immediately to stop the growth of dangerous bacteria. One takes it in juice or water every little while. *Warning:* if a doctor must resort to an antibiotic, which is sometimes necessary to avoid serious weakness, yogurt or acidophilus *must* be taken simultaneously or as soon as possible. Antibiotics do indeed kill tenacious germs in the body, but they also kill the friendly intestinal flora. European doctors understand this and prescribe some form of soured milk or acidophilus simultaneously with the antibiotic. Otherwise constipation and an under par feeling may continue indefinitely.

One of the causes of diarrhea can be intestinal parasites or worms. A very recent report[14] states that hundreds of Americans and others who have drunk tap water in the Soviet Union have come home with an intestinal parasite infection, called *Giardasis*. This ailment differs from other diarrheas picked up by foreign travelers, in that it does not begin until the traveler returns home and can last for months. Although it is true that certain drugs can kill this and other types of parasites (in this case, the drugs atabrine or flagyl) most people who take worm- or parasite-killing drugs wish they hadn't. It can be a horrific experience, believe me.

There is another natural remedy, used by scores of medical doctors,[15] which has controlled diarrhea and dysentery of various origins as well as routing parasites. This is garlic, whether fresh, in powder, tablet, or perle form. It is a powerful, natural, effective but harmless antibiotic, and aids digestion. Eleanor Roosevelt even took it to improve her memory! It is available in tablets or perles at health stores. "Social" garlic, which is odorless, is also available, although whether it is as effective as the natural, I do not know.

As for supplements, the late Dr. Tom Spies, of Hillman Hospital, Birmingham, Alabama, treated diarrhea—which in some cases is an early symptom of pellagra—with niacin, a B vitamin.

Diarrhea was often reversed within a week. Adelle Davis stated that she had seen many cases of diarrhea which had lasted for years clear up in a day or so with a daily natural source of B vitamins (brewer's yeast and liver) plus 100 mg. of niacinamide, which does not cause skin flushing. She added that Vitamin B-6, folic acid, magnesium and calcium are also necessary for those prone to diarrhea.[16]

The old diet during or following diarrhea was usually tea and toast. Avoiding solid foods, drinking bland liquids, water and weak teas, followed by bland solid foods (nothing raw) was the order of the day. No longer! Adelle Davis advised to get those missing nutrients, especially the minerals, back into the body as fast as possible.

She wrote, "It has been found that far greater quantities of all nutrients are retained if large meals are eaten instead of small ones, even though hearty meals may make the diarrhea temporarily worse." The foods need not be smooth or low in residue, she said, but merely as rich as possible in vitamins, minerals, oils and proteins. . . . Yogurt and acidophilus should be heavily relied upon, as well as digestive enzymes with bile, hydrochloric acid and lecithin until the putrefactive bacteria are under control.[16]

As for allergic diarrhea, watch the effects of what you eat (see chapter on allergics).

To remove sprays and other toxic poisons from food, use the following *safe* water bath to cleanse them. (Strawberries in my area have been doused with arsenic. Bananas are gassed, so any suspicious foods should be treated):

Use ½ teaspoon of Clorox to one gallon of water. In this low concentration it has been tested for safety for ten years.

For thin-skinned fruits and vegetables, place in this bath for ten minutes. Root vegetables and heavy-skinned fruits, including bananas with skins, require fifteen to twenty minutes. Make a new batch of the mixture for each category. Transfer to a fresh water bath for ten to fifteen minutes before using or refrigerating food.

There is absolutely no bleach aftertaste. Fruits and vegetables actually keep longer; wilted ones become crisper. One couple driving from Texas to California several times a year carried their own food with them. Before they learned about this method of treatment they had to discard the fresh food before they reached home. After treating the food by this method in Texas, it was still firm and fresh by the time they reached California. Other friends who travel in foreign countries take a small bottle of this same Clorox and add one drop to every glass of drinking water for decontamination. They have never acquired diarrhea, whereas others around them were stricken.

A final remedy for diarrhea has been handed down by our great grandparents: blackberry wine. One or two 2-oz. glasses of the wine for adults, and smaller amounts for babies, have been said to stop the diarrhea in an hour. A pleasant remedy, worth a try!

REFERENCES
(See *Bibliography* for fuller details.)

1. Irwin Stone, *The Healing Factor: Vitamin C Against Disease*.
2. John E. Eichenlaub, M.D., *A Minnesota Doctor's Home Remedies for Common and Uncommon Ailments*.
3. D. C. Jarvis, M.D., *Folk Medicine*.
4. Linda Clark, *Secrets of Health and Beauty*.
5. *Consumers' Report*, Feb. 26, 1974.
6. Write for information about *Bentonite* to Veico Products, Natick, Mass. 01670.
7. *Journal of Pediatrics*, June, 1950.
8. *Prevention*, October, 1965.
9. *Journal of the Michigan Medical School*, 36: 40, 1937.
10. *Bulletin of the Biological Science Foundation, Ltd.*, March–April, 1956.
11. *The Lancet*, March 6, 1954.
12. *The New York Times*, July 4, 1971.
13. *Post Graduate Medicine*, July 1956.
14. *The New York Times*, March 11, 1974.
15. J. I. Rodale and Staff, *Encyclopedia of Common Diseases*.
16. Adelle Davis, *Let's Get Well*.

13: DIVERTICULOSIS, DIVERTICULITIS

Diverticulosis may seem to be a comparative newcomer to the list of health disturbances. Actually, many people may have suffered from this malady for years without knowing it. Its discovery is becoming increasingly common.

What is It?

Diverticula are small balloon-like protuberances on the intestinal walls of the colon. They can range from the size of a pea to the size of a thimble, but regardless of size can become lodging places for decaying particles of food or fecal matter. These small pouches of sewage deposits can breed putrefying bacteria. They may later become inflamed, and cause irritation as well as pain. If this stage is reached, the disturbance is know as diverticulitis (inflammation of the diverticula).

In spite of a good diet, people, even animals, sometimes develop anemia as a result of diverticular disease because the putrefactive bacteria gobble up the B vitamin, folic acid, and prevent it from reaching the blood. Other problems, both intestinal and general, may develop due to the increase of toxins generated by this condition.

What Causes It?

There are several theories to explain the cause of diverticular disease. One theory is that gas cannot be expelled normally and is diverted against the intestinal walls, thus creating the small thin-walled pouches. Another theory is that when waste matter in the intestines is scanty, intense contraction required to expel it puts great pressure on the intestinal muscles, causing the pouches to form. In other words, the expulsion of gas or waste is diverted against the intestinal walls of the sigmoid colon (above the rectum), creating the little sacs which are called *diverticula,* a name which comes from the word "diverted."

There is some speculation that muscle walls may also be in a weakened condition due to lack of protein or the minerals, potassium and manganese, both involved in muscle integrity, and perhaps even a deficiency of certain types of calcium which can help to prevent cell disintegration. Incidentally, the presence of diverticulosis is usually established by means of X-rays.

What is The Solution?

Many physicians advise surgery to remove the diverticula, but Adelle Davis wisely pointed out that the surgical removal of old diverticula does not prevent the formation of new ones. She believes that correction and prevention by nutritional means is best.[1] Her suggestions include:

Improving digestion.

Decreasing gas formation.

Building stronger intestinal walls to resist ballooning.

Relieving stress to avoid tension building up in the body which includes the intestines. (Adelle believed it is as possible to "blow your intestines" as it is to "blow your top.")

What nutrients can be used to fulfill these requirements? Hydrochloric acid[2] oftens relieves gas from undigested protein. Other digestive enzymes, in combination, for digesting starches, fats and proteins are usually available from health stores.

Vitamins can help, too. Vitamin E is a well-known muscle strengthener (witness its reported effect upon the heart, a muscle).[3] The B vitamins are needed, not only to provide the folic acid, but to prevent stress and strengthen nerves. Vitamin C, of course, is considered an efficient detoxifier. It is never wise to pick only one or two vitamins to alleviate *any* condition. Vitamin deficiencies rarely occur singly even though the effects of lack of one may show up first. In nature, they all appear and work together.

This applies to minerals, too, which are a must in diverticular disease. Potassium or manganese, as well as calcium and magnesium can play a part in muscular as well as nerve health.[3] It is better to be fortified with a source of all minerals, perhaps from kelp, possibly stepping up those which are in greatest need, separately.

What Diet is Best?

For quite some time there was controversy about a diverticulosis diet. Most orthodox doctors long maintained that a bland diet completely devoid of roughage should be followed to the letter. I know people who, when invited to a meal, warn the poor hostess, "I can't eat salads, raw vegetables or fruits, or *any* roughage due to my diverticulosis. Doctor's orders!"

Adelle Davis disagreed. She says, "Because foods supplying cellulose, unrefined starches and natural roughage support the growth of the *valuable* bacteria or intestinal flora (which helps to vanquish the putrefactive bacteria), the diet generally recommended for diverticulosis appears to be the very one to be avoided."

Many doctors are beginning to agree. One of these, George C. Thosteson, M.D., who writes a syndicated newspaper medical column, admits, to his credit, "It was formerly assumed that roughage should be kept to a minimum in the diet for diverticulosis. Now it appears that this is not the wisest course. Patients are better off with a moderate amount of bulk since there is less stress when the colon is comfortably filled."

Two British physicians have gone still further. Drs. Neil S.

Painter and Denis T. Burkitt have reported that 85% of patients using more bulk, especially unprocessed bran, in the diet, were relieved of symptoms of diverticulosis.[4] (See also the reference to the work of these doctors in chapter on constipation.)

Dr. Thosteson does not believe in overdoing the low-residue thing. He points out that there are differences in bran—some coarser than others, thus more irritating, which he feels should be avoided along with seeds and vegetables with tough hulls, such as corn. He does not believe that orange juice should be strained, nor other fruit pulp omitted. He recommends the use of psyllium seed and agar products for providing nonirritating bulk. Many other doctors, however, recommend the softer forms of bran (such as bran flakes) and report excellent results.

There is another problem among those who are both nutritional converts and diverticulosis patients, as the following letter written to me shows:

"Inasmuch as I am troubled with diverticulitis and take about 30 supplements, or I get an attack, I have to hammer them all into powder form.

"I wish the vitamin/mineral industries could realize the millions of persons who have diverticulosis so that they would make the supplements in powder form, enclosed in capsules."

Although it is simple to powder vitamin and mineral tablets in one of those little electric grinders used for grains and seeds (at health and hardware stores), a method which is easier than hammering, still this is a point well taken. Supplement manufacturers, please take note!

Meanwhile there is a nutritional help for use in cleansing residue from the intestinal tract, as well as in preventing further breeding of the putrefactive bacteria. Nutritionists recommend liberal amounts of yogurt and acidophilus (the latter, which is stronger and more active, is available at health stores) to help increase the beneficial intestinal flora or bacteria. These products also help to combat gas, indigestion, constipation, and keep the intestines in healthy condition.

Finally, digestive enzymes, which include hydrochloric acid and other digestants, may be a key to relief from diverticulosis.

A nutritional consultant shared the following case histories with me:

A postman was suffering from diverticulosis and fear. His brother had suffered from a "bursted intestine" and he was afraid the same thing would happen to him. Although his doctor had scheduled surgery for him within six weeks, he was in the meantime suffering from his condition which was intensified by his necessity to stay on his feet to keep his job as a postman. The nutritionist, after questioning him, suggested digestive enzymes. The postman stated later that two tablets had provided relief within an hour. He continued taking the digestive aids, and reported that his trouble seemed to have disappeared. When his doctor rechecked him, prior to the planned operation, the examination showed no signs of diverticulosis at all!

—A woman who had been going to a doctor for over a year, with no results, obtained complete relief in two weeks with digestive enzymes.

—A man had suffered from diverticulitis for forty years, without relief even though he had been through a university hospital clinic twice. Their only suggestion was sedation, which relieved but did not cure the symptoms. Digestive enzymes plus 3 or 4 ounces of aloe vera once to twice daily provided complete relief.

Again, one remedy may work for some and not others. You may need to try various remedies mentioned in this chapter until you find the one that works for you.

REFERENCES
(See *Bibliography* for fuller details.)

1. Adelle Davis, *Let's Get Well*.
2. Linda Clark, *Secrets of Health and Beauty*.
3. Linda Clark, *Know Your Nutrition*.
4. *British Medical Journal*, May 22, 1971.

14: EPILEPSY

There is a lot of twiddle-twaddle about epilepsy. Just as one swallow does not make a summer, neither does one convulsion decree epilepsy. As most people who are conversant with true epilepsy know, there are two general types of convulsions or "seizures." One is called *Petit Mal,* borrowed from the French, and meaning "little sickness." The other type is known as *Grand Mal,* also from the French, meaning "big sickness."

Petit Mal is more common in children than in adults; may occur frequently, as often as a hundred or more times daily; last only a few seconds, and be no more noticeable than a slight hesitation, or a rhythmic twitching of eyelids or eyebrows. A child may fall but will get up again immediately. *Petit Mal* is usually worse in the morning, with fewer attacks appearing during the day. This type also becomes less frequent as a child grows older.

Grand Mal, on the other hand, may be characterized by the patient becoming unconscious, falling, possibly with saliva or froth appearing on his lips. His muscles may twitch violently, or tighten into a spasm of convulsion for a minute or two. The patient may bite his tongue seriously unless something is placed between his teeth. Usually a true epileptic, or even a pseudo, may have warning of a forthcoming attack. A strange sensation in the stomach, a dizzy feeling, or even an imagined unpleasant odor are some clues which may give a preview of the coming seizure. There may be a memory lapse after the seizure has passed; the patient may feel drowsy, or he may fall asleep and sleep for hours.

What is True Epilepsy?

True epilepsy is a disorder of the nervous system involving the rhythm of electrical discharges from the brain, resulting in sudden and recurring episodes of unconsciousness. As previously noted, this varies from a slight lapse in awareness, as in *Petit Mal*, to a major loss of consciousness and convulsive movements, as in *Grand Mal*.

What Causes Epilepsy?

Some children are admittedly born epileptics, with brain damage, but the number is comparatively small. Doctors diagnose epilepsy by means of a machine known as an electroencephalograph. Electrodes are attached to the head and the instrument records the electrical brain currents in a graph, known as an EEG (electroencephalogram). But this test, even when coupled with muscle biopsies, can be misleading. Results of such diagnoses can show *identical* patterns in true epilepsy that are also evident with a deficiency of certain nutritional substances affecting the brain.

Therefore doctors may be too quick in concluding that a convulsion has been caused by true epilepsy. Actually a convulsion can be caused by a dozen other problems.

Allergies are a major cause. Hal M. Davison, M.D., reported that both *Petit Mal* and *Grand Mal* were produced five times in one patient by eating cauliflower and were relieved when the food was withdrawn. Other patients had "epileptic" attacks from various foods including eggs, cereals, milk and mushrooms. Yet when Dr. Davison sent a questionnaire to 1,494 allergy specialists, asking for opinions on the possible result of "epileptic type attacks" from allergies, only 207 answered, and with such responses as "not suspected" or "never occurred to me," or "overlooked."[1]

Hypoglycemia has been found to be another factor in producing "epileptic" type convulsions by those late respected pioneers, Drs. E. W. Abrahamson and Seale Harris. Even the lay public is becoming aware that blackouts can be a common symptom of hypoglycemia.

Convulsions can also occur when the calcium drops to a low level in the blood. Another cause of convulsions, originally diagnosed as epilepsy, has been traced to exposure to the insecticide, dieldrin.

John M. Ellis, M.D. found that a deficiency in Vitamin B-6 caused by excessively heated commercial milk formulas produced convulsions in babies.[2]

Dr. John Ott has publicized "TV epilepsy," which he found common in children due to the flickering light of TV, especially when viewed from the side, rather than at least six feet away and in front of the screen. Children exhibited other serious symptoms including hyperactivity, headache, nervousness, fatigue, loss of sleep and vomiting in direct ratio to the number of hours spent before a TV.[3] *Organic Consumer Report*[4] published this letter as an example of one case of "TV epilepsy:"

"Three years ago our two-year-old son was watching TV while I was preparing his lunch, which he usually ate while watching his favorite program.

"As I set his tray down in front of him, I noticed that his eyes were rolled back in his head, and he sat frozen. He didn't respond to his name, although I shook him and tried to arouse him. Then he started turning blue. I did all of the usual things to keep him breathing while a neighbor drove us to the doctor, who worked over him for two hours.

"Our little boy was weak and listless for a few days, during which time TV seemed a godsend, to keep him inside. A few weeks passed and he had another attack, but this time I had a prescription tranquilizer on hand and used it according to the doctor's instructions. He quieted down, slept soundly and then awoke in about two hours. He started running through the house like a wild animal, yelling and hitting things. We were frantic and the doctor recommended hospitalization for diagnostic purposes.

"In a children's hospital a battery of tests was done, including an encephalograph. Finally the doctors old us that our son had epilepsy and would have to be on medication *for life*, at increasing potencies; he warned that he should not ride his bicycle, or later, play football.

"Every time we gave him the drug prescribed, it had the effect of overstimulating him, and he would yell and cry and run wildly. Finally we decided to skip medication every other day and see what happened. He calmed down on those days, so then we started skipping medication two days, then three, etc. Before long we discontinued it altogether, gradually cutting it down.

"Now we know that our son does not have epilepsy, although that was the medical verdict of the term of 'experts'. None of them seem to know what did happen to him to cause those spells. Have you ever hear of anything similar?"

COMMENT (by *O.C.R.*): a growing number of children in the U.S. and Europe have been diagnosed as epileptic. When they failed to respond satisfactorily to drugs and tranquilizers commonly used and prescribed, many doctors began to question. Apparently greater numbers were afflicted in Europe, where the "disease" was first diagnosed as "TV Epilepsy," than in the U.S., which stimulated researchers to find out why. In certain types of epilepsy one of the things that can bring on an attack is flickering light. The viewing of TV can bring on such an attack.

I have personally witnessed several misdiagnoses of epilepsy. One was a young boy who had had convulsions from time to time. The parents were reluctant to use drugs and, on a hunch, took their son to a chiropractor who found a definite misalignment in the spine in the neck area. The atlas was found out of place, as proved by X-ray. When this was corrected by an adjustment, the convulsions disappeared, but not permanently. Every time there was a recurrence, the atlas again was found to be out of alignment. This apparently was caused by nerve pressure in the neck which interfered with circulation to the brain, leading to the convulsions. The chiropractor questioned the boy and his parents. He learned two things: the boy had had a head injury a year previous to the onset of the convulsions as a result of being accidentally hit by a baseball bat, and more recently he had let his hair grow long like his friends, and the chiropractor noticed that the boy often jerked his head to one side to get his long hair out of his eyes. This apparently triggered the atlas musculature which had been seriously weakened by the baseball bat injury. After the boy had his hair cut, and returned regularly for check-ups to the chiropractor for *prevention* of misalignment, the convulsions became less and less frequent, as the neck muscles became stronger and began to hold the atlas in place. However, a disturbing episode followed.

The boy went to a Boy Scout camp, and due to some unknown cause had a convulsion while there. The camp doctor phoned the parents and demanded that they come for their son immediately. Otherwise he threatened to take him to a hospital and start drug treatment for epilepsy. The parents did take the boy home, refused drugs and hospitalization, and returned to the chiropractor who, as usual, found the atlas out of place. With correction by adjustment and continued regular check-ups, the convulsions eventually ceased without resort to drugs.

Another case I observed was that of a young married woman who, with her husband, had returned to the United States from a tropical foreign country where they had been stationed for several years. After their return, the wife suddenly developed convulsions. She was taken to a doctor and a clinic, which established the diagnosis of epilepsy as the result of an EEG. A report was sent to the State Department of Motor Vehicles by the doctor, as required by the state, threatening her status as a driver.

Meanwhile she was referred by a friend to a nutritionally

oriented M.D. This doctor found that she had intestinal parasites, a common occurrence in the country where the couple had
been living. When these were eliminated by herbal means[5] and
nutritional substances given liberally, the convulsions ceased,
never to return. Since there were no further seizures, her
driver's license was reinstated and her so-called misdiagnosed
"epilepsy" is now a closed chapter.

Pros and Cons of Drugs

There is an estimate from medical authorities that from two to
four million Americans have some form of epilepsy, and that
with the use of modern drugs, half of those afflicted can be completely free of seizures; another one third can obtain partial control of their epileptic attacks.

Here is a vote for the use of an epilepsy drug, as written to
Ann Landers in her nationally syndicated column, December 5,
1970:

Dear Ann Landers:

I am a normal 15-year-old girl. When I say normal I mean I look like a
15-year-old girl, I act like a 15-year-old girl and I have all the desires
and dreams of a 15-year-old girl. The only way in which I am different
is that I am an epileptic.

I have the Epilepsy Foundation to thank for educating me so that I now
live a fear-free life. I have learned from their booklets to hold my head
up and to help other epileptics. I have also learned not to be ashamed of
my affliction.

It is estimated that one out of every 100 people have epilepsy. This
means about two million in the United States. And don't forget—for
every epileptic, three or four members of his family are involved in his
illness. They should understand the nature of epilepsy and know what
to do in case of a seizure.

I have not had a seizure in years, thanks to dilantin, a marvelous drug
which has changed the lives of millions. Please, Ann Landers, print the

address of the Epilepsy Foundation and urge interested people to write for free literature. They also have films for groups who wish to understand. God bless you for the good you do.

(Signed) "One of Two Million."[6]

On the other hand, here is a letter from a man, written to *me*:
"Several years ago I had a series of memory lapses, usually the first thing in the morning. A neurologist prescribed large doses of dilantin which I took with the assurance that there would be no side effects. Later, I learned that the drug inactivates folic acid. I stopped taking the drug and discovered I had acquired degeneration of the retina, for which four opthalmologists told me there was no cure. So, though I stopped the drug, now it is too late."

Dilantin and mesantoin are used for *Grand Mal,* and triodone for *Petit Mal.* New ones may be added from time to time. Side effects, sometimes very serious ones, may occur from such drugs, and this necessitates careful supervision by physicians.

Before turning to drugs, you should know of the beneficial effects of certain nutritional substances used by some *medical doctors* for convulsions, even for those considered true epileptics. More than twenty-five years ago, the late Tom Spies, M.D., gave Vitamin B-6 with excellent results to epileptics. More recently, babies, fed a well-known formula, had repeated seizures. The administrations of B-6 stopped the convulsions and the EEGs became normal within minutes.[7]

David Baird Coursin, M.D., of the Research Institute at St. Joseph Hospital, Lancaster, Pennsylvania, established by EEG the changes in patients' brainwaves resulting from a deficiency of Vitamin B-6. Among other case histories submitted by Dr. Coursin is one patient, who, after an injection of B-6, had no further convulsions, exhibited an improvement of brainwave forms and rapidly became normal. Dr. Coursin points out that the B-6 needs vary with the individual. For some patients small amounts of the vitamin will be sufficient to reverse their symptoms; others will require larger amounts. Oral doses may suffice for some; injections may be needed for others.[8] Adelle Davis cautioned, however, that if large amounts of Vitamin B-6 are given, the other B vitamins, found in the entire complex or family, should also be given.

Another wonder worker for true epileptics, whether *Petit Mal* or *Grand Mal,* is magnesium. Adelle Davis reported one study of thirty epileptic children, formerly on anticonvulsant drugs, who were given 450 milligrams of magnesium daily, and drugs were no longer needed. Another case she reported is that of a 13-year-old boy who had been an epileptic for ten years. He was both depressed and showed signs of mental retardation. Drugs could not prevent his seizures. Magnesium, however, did the trick. He became mentally alert and his epilepsy disappeared.[7]

Adelle Davis stated that she had planned nutrition programs for at least fifty epileptic patients, all of whom, to her knowledge, had remained free of the illness, without the use of drugs. Both B-6 and magnesium were incorporated into their nutritional diets.[7] Vitamin E has also been responsible for reversal of convulsions in true epilepsy.[9]

Exact dosages of these and other vitamins for epileptics, for both children and adults, may be found in Dr. Paavo Airola's book, *How to Get Well.*[10]

The Orientals have other successful health treatments up their sleeves in addition to acupuncture. Herbal therapy has been one of their health tools for centuries. In the book, *Healing Ourselves,* the author, Naboru Muramoto, gives the case history of a woman, who, after injuring her spine at the age of thirteen, had suffered from epileptic seizures for twenty-two years. She was given, at that late date, the Oriental Day Lily Tea, considered excellent for the nervous system. She took it for sixty days only. She no longer needs the medicine prescribed by a doctor and has had no recurrence of the convulsions.[11]

Homeopathic substances, chosen for each individual case by homeopathic physicians, have also worked wonders. A fourteen-year-old boy had suffered from epilepsy for ten years, with the diagnosis confirmed by an EEG. The boy was considered incurable; he suffered from fifteen to thirty epileptic sei-zures daily, during waking hours as well as sleep. The homeopathic substance *Silicea* was given in gradually ascending potencies by a homeopathic physician, and the boy has not had a single seizure in three years.[12]

What Epilepsy is Not

Many patients, as well as their families, suffer from a feeling of shame resulting from true epilepsy or epileptic-like symptoms. Other children at school make fun of the victim, or regard as an outcast the one who suffers untold agony and the fear of possi-ble convulsions or social condemnation, or both. Yet even true epilepsy is not related to insanity, does not lead to delinquency, vice or crime. It is not hereditary. It is not "catching." It can be controlled, as you have seen, and is no more to be ashamed of than diabetes or some other affliction.

Suggestions for Doctors and Patients

Comments of misdiagnoses of epileptics in this discussion are not meant as condemnation of doctors, who no doubt do their duty as they see it. The plea, however, is for less superficial diag-nosis of the disorder, leaving the poor patient with a life stigma of a label of epilepsy (true or false) which can color his entire future, in social, business and employment, even marriage as-sociations, and thus ruin him as an individual. I urge you, there-fore, to look first for a possible nutritional deficiency disease, or some other natural cause (i.e., parasites, injury, allergy, hypo-glycemia, etc.), and aim to correct, as well as prevent, the symptoms rather than mask them by drugs merely because they may seem to be the easiest way out. Avoid unnecessary publicity and consider your patient with compassion.

REFERENCES

(See *Bibliography* for fuller details.)

1. *Quarterly Review of Allergy and Applied Immunology*, June, 1952.

2. John M. Ellis, M.D., "A Review of Vitamin B-6," *Natural Food & Farming*, June, 1974.

3. *Time* magazine, November 6, 1964.

4. *Organic Consumer Report*, May 17, 1966.

5. Alan H. Nittler, *A New Breed of Doctor*.

6. Address: The Epilepsy Foundation, 1729 F Street, N.W., Washington, D. C. 20006.

7. Adelle Davis, *Let's Get Well*.

8. John M. Ellis, M.D., with James Presley, *Vitamin B-6: The Doctor's Report*.

9. J. I. Rodale and Staff, *Encyclopedia of Common Diseases*.

10. Paavo Airola, Ph.D., N.D., *How To Get Well*.

11. Naboru Nuramoto, *Healing Ourselves*. (Also contains addresses of sources of Oriental teas.)

12. *The Layman Speaks*, p. 140, June, 1974.

For information on homeopathic physicians in your area, write: National Center for Homeopathy, Suite 506, 6231 Leesburg Pike, Falls Church, Va. 22041.

15: FATIGUE

Many people are tired all of the time. They drag from one task to another, not realizing that this chronic fatigue is not usually really necessary, or that energy can be improved with a minimum of effort, providing they know what to do about it. And what exactly *can* be done about it? That is what this chapter is about.

There are several causes of chronic fatigue. Everybody already knows that temporary fatigue can stem from overworking and underresting, so we won't belabor these obvious conclusions. Nearly everyone has to work overtime now and then, perhaps sacrificing rest or sleep for that particular occasion. A man may have a deadline work assignment. A woman may have to clean the whole house for the unexpected arrival of a guest. A student may have to work long hours to get ready for an exam. These are common emergencies, and though tiring, the lost rest can probably be made up later. But a specific character trait, compulsiveness, can create *continuous* fatigue for many people. And this must be stopped in its tracks!

Are You Compulsive?

Many housewives and more than a few businessmen feel on a regular basis that they cannot relax until they finish up everything that needs to be done, *at one time.* These people are usually perfectionists, tense, and cannot rest until they get the last detail on their list done *now,* no matter how weary they are. They drive themselves relentlessly to finish their self-imposed goal before they sink exhausted into the nearest chair, feeling triumphant and not a little smug and virtuous. Witness the housewife, about to take off for the family vacation, who insists she cannot leave until the house is cleaned. Fine. A clean house is a joy to return to after a vacation. But this does not mean adding a spring cleaning, changing the furniture around, painting the back porch and sorting out the attic while she is about it! Nor does the businessman have to pick that prevacation time to answer all of his piled-up correspondence, already months old, or suddenly book appointments with people he had been planning to see but putting off for the past year. Two more weeks won't make that much difference. When he returns from his vacation he will be feeling more fit and ready to discharge those accumulated tasks he couldn't face earlier, with greater dispatch.

A psychiatrist once told me, "A typical compulsive person is one who is rushing out the door, already late for an appointment, but *has* to stop to straighten the rug he tripped over before leaving."

In other words, if you are compulsive, *let something go.* Adopt a mañana, or laissez-faire or "So What" attitude. You will experience less fatigue and tension, enjoy life more and be far easier to live with. And you may even get more done in the long run. As my Pennsylvania Dutch grandmother often said, "The hurrieder I go, the behinder I get."

Fatigue can also result from unresolved emotional problems. When a satisfactory solution is found, the feeling of carrying a burden, often accompanied by great weariness or fatigue, usually clears.

Try it!

Another cause of chronic fatigue, which makes you feel like a clock run down, is poor circulation. This is easy to remedy: merely add some exercise on a daily basis. Housewives, or even men who are physically active, will insist that they already get too much exercise. Oh, no they don't! I don't mean movement, I mean *exercise*. A woman may clean her house or do other household chores and go through movements, but not exercise. She may be tense because she hates housework and this tension stifles rather than encourages good circulation. Consequently she is more tired than refreshed after finishing her daily chores, be it cleaning, washing, ironing or whatever.

As an example, I have told elsewhere of a woman who helped me weekly with my own house cleaning. She was young, had a family, and was always tired. Before she came to my house, or that of others each day, she had to tidy up her own house after getting her husband and children off to work and school. By the time she arrived she was exhausted. When I asked her if she took regular exercise, she looked at me as if I had flipped. So I explained the tension concept and suggested that she do a few push-ups, or other calisthenics plus deep breathing exercises each morning before she started her day.

She returned a week later looking and feeling like a different person. She said that the ten minutes of daily exercise had limbered her up and given her extra energy which carried her through the whole day, a fact she would have never believed until she tried it.

If calisthenics bore you, try something you enjoy: walking, bicycling, swimming, bowling, gardening, golf or tennis, but make it regular. You will find that it gives you more zest.

Sedentary workers should get on their feet whenever possible, stand instead of sit, and walk instead of ride, at every opportunity.

What Else Causes Fatigue?

However, perhaps you are not compulsive, don't overwork, do

get enough exercise and rest, have no unresolved emotional problems, have excellent circulation and are still tired all the time. If so, you may be suffering from low octane fuel. Your body engine may be underfunctioning because it is not receiving "premium" food. At least this is the cause of lack of energy in millions of Americans, according to Drs. E. Cheraskin and W.M. Ringsdorf, Jr.[1] They state that the typical American may skip breakfast, lunch or dinner. Or if he does eat these meals, the breakfast consists of coffee with sugar, a "Danish" or a donut. Lunch is usually a sandwich on white bread plus more coffee or a soft drink. Dinner may be better balanced, but not enough to atone for the omissions of the earlier meals, or the fact that all eating during the day has been laced together with coffee breaks, usually including sweets of some kind.

This kind of food, which is usually processed, devitalized, full of artificial additives, and considered anything but premium quality for body building or sustaining, has been found to be the main fare of those who feel chronically tired and suffer from irritability, headaches, insomnia, overweight, and "nerves." Drs. Cheraskin and Ringsdorf equate such food with undernutrition, or malnutrition, and the FDA won't admit that this is the bulk of the food supplied to us Americans. Nor do they admit that it hurts us. The Department of Agriculture, on the other hand, has conducted surveys which prove that such food is common and *is* producing widespread undernutrition or malnutrition.[2]

The average American's food has been found inadequate in protein, vitamin and mineral content, and high in carbohydrates (sugars and starches) which lead to obesity, nervousness, tiredness and a host of other complaints so prevalent today. Why? We can again liken the cause to a sluggish car engine. Without a continuous supply of proper fuel, the car's ignition, transmission, carburetor, and general performance will gradually grind to a halt. In the body, the organs and glands which run it must have their equivalent in proper fuel to provide energy and rev up the body motor to top performance. Ask those you have noticed to have recent, increased sustained pep what their secret is, and nine times out of ten they will tell you that they have upped their vitamins, minerals, and health foods.

What Not to Do

The others who have only a burst of energy now and then, are still no doubt depending on crutches to get them through life: aspirin, pep pills, tranquilizers and other drugs; alcohol; coffee; smoking, and sweets. You probably know by this time that if you suddenly feel tired, eating some sugar or drinking a cup of coffee will indeed give you a temporary energy lift, since it raises your blood sugar. But this is soon followed by a downward plunge of energy, leaving you feeling worse then before, calling for a repetition of more coffee and sweets or alcohol, creating a continuous and vicious circle. The result? Illnesses that are affecting millions today: low blood sugar (hypoglycemia) or alcoholism, or both. These conditions can lead to real trouble like blackouts, and sometimes a complete breakdown of the body.

How crazy to be a sheep, doing what everyone else is doing, when by making only a few changes, you can avoid all this and tiredness, too. Adding "premium" food to your way of life may result in a surprising improvement in your energy and make life worth living. Don't take my word for it. Try it for yourself, just as more and more people are already learning to do every day. You couldn't pay them to return to their old ways of eating and that horrible feeling of being half alive.

How to Eat for Energy

1. Forget those three squares a day. They probably aren't squares, anyway, but unbalanced or at least inadequate. It is better to eat oftener and less, but make that "less" count and really do something for yourself besides just filling up. Eat health foods that build you up, not empty fuels that break you down.

2. Substitute protein for sweets at every opportunity. At home the housewife can rely on her own refrigerator for a snack, but there should only be sensible snacks in it. If you don't buy junk food and bring it home, it won't be there to tempt you. Use chunks of cheese, or a few nuts as nibbles. A piece of raw

fruit or carrot or celery contains free vitamins and minerals. Or make a protein powder drink with fruit juice for breakfast or lunch and you shouldn't feel tired for hours.

3. If you want a quick, fatigue-routing snack, eat a little fat. You heard me, I said *fat*! This belief that eating fat will make you fat is stuff-and-nonsense. Researchers have learned that some fat is needed to make your gall bladder work (a lack of fat has caused gall stones)[3], as well as to give your hair and skin some sheen. There is the report by Adelle Davis of those who could not lose weight until they added two tablespoons of vegetable oil to their diet. Presto! off went the pounds.[3]

Another thing about eating fat—it staves off hunger as well as fatigue for hours. Either add a bit of vegetable oil to your protein drink before you blend it (you will never know it's there) or add more oil to your salad at mealtime and drink the remains from the bowl. Or, if you want a snack only, take a spoonful of peanut butter straight, or stuff a stalk of celery with it.

4. If you are at the office, cut down on your coffee intake. One Master of Ceremonies of a well-known TV talk show has admitted to his audience that he developed hypoglycemia from the cups and cups of coffee which were constantly served him during rehearsals. One cup of coffee in the morning will probably not finish you off, particularly if you grind it yourself and filter drip it, but additional cups throughout the day can eventually lead to severe fatigue associated with hypoglycemia. Take your own decaffeinated coffee with you to work, or go English-style and brew a cup of tea which is allowed on most hypoglycemic diets. Some people prefer herb tea and take along their own tea bags.

People who habitually feel tired and weak, as well as shaky and irritable during the day are usually hypoglycemics, suffering from low blood sugar which needs a boost with not only some protein, but frequent, small meals to shore up their energy. By eating some sensible food their pep seems to return miraculously, and if protein or fat are included, that pep can last for several hours.

Even if you do have a cup of coffee, you can cut down on part of the trouble by having some protein (instead of a sweet) with it, to prevent that sudden dip in blood sugar. This will obviate part of that tiredness, at least. When I had my own radio show, I took along hulled, high protein sunflower seeds and passed them around to the staff who were constantly guzzling coffee at the coffee machine. One secretary, said, "Since you brought those sunflower seeds, I don't have four o'clock slump anymore."

Even popcorn, which is a nutritious grain, is better than sweets, and most people love it. You can bring it to the office already popped, or if you have a hot plate, pop it on the spot in one of those little pop-it gadgets available at grocery stores. You need not stand the cost for these nutritious additions to office coffee-break snacks either. Pool money for them and take turns supplying and making them available to your coworkers. The idea will soon catch on as people begin to feel better.

5. This brings up cocktail parties and what to substitute for that drink you really don't want or shouldn't have. One nationally known artist who exhibits her work regularly invites her friends to a preview the first day of the exhibit. Refreshments are served. Since she believes in nutrition, these refreshments are both nutritious and delicious. She makes her own tiny open-faced sandwiches of various spreads on natural whole grain, thinly sliced bread, and serves exotic nuts and usually no sweets at all. She offers champagne to those who want it and imported natural white grapejuice to those who don't. The glasses in which both beverages are served are identical and no one knows who is drinking which. Even if they did, they couldn't care less. Her friends are emancipated people who are absolutely indifferent to keeping up with the Joneses. They consider it smart and chic to do their own thing and they look and feel better for it.

What Supplements Help Prevent Fatigue?

A deficiency in certain vitamins and minerals have been found to be a factor in fatigue. Many people are resorting to the use of pep pills and tranquilizers. This is sad because such drugs merely mask and perpetuate tiredness, not correct it. The entire Vitamin B complex protects nerves and increases energy since it helps to feed, nourish and regulate glands, which are the machinery of the body.

Foods rich in the B vitamins are liver, brewer's yeast, wheat germ, rice polishings, etc. Brewer's yeast contains a minimum of ten B vitamins as well as eighteen minerals and sixteen protein factors (amino acids), and has raised the energy level of many people in a surprisingly short time. Taking some of it in juice or water, preferably just before you become too tired, can give you the lift of a cup of coffee, but lasts hours instead of minutes, as coffee does.[4]

Liver is another energizer. For those of you who insist upon becoming vegetarians, remember that George Bernard Shaw, also a vegetarian, finally was forced to resort to liver injections, which he called his "medicine," in order to remain vital. Desiccated liver in tablet form is easier for most people to include in their diet and it has been found extremely helpful in preventing tiredness. B. M. Ershoff, M.D. tested three groups of swimming rats. Two groups were fed other diets; the third, desiccated liver. The first two groups became fatigued early in the test, whereas those fed desiccated liver were still swimming vigorously without fatigue at the end of the experiment.[5]

Other vitamins play specific roles in fatigue in connection with various ailments. By correcting the deficiency, the fatigue will vanish.

Minerals are important, too. According to the late Charles Northen, "In the absence of minerals, vitamins have no function."[6]

What Physical Conditions Cause Fatigue?

Anemia is a No. 1 ailment leading to fatigue. It is known as a "tired blood" disturbance, and iron and Vitamin B-12 are usually the most common nutrients recommended by doctors. However, there are other deficiencies often involved in anemia, including Vitamin B-6, Vitamin E, and folic acid. Although many suffer from deficiency of iron, trouble can actually result from taking the wrong kind of iron, or too much of it.[7] (For details, see Chapter Four on Anemia.)

My own favorite iron product is a food iron which includes powdered, edible hemoglobin, dried yeast, desiccated whole liver, natural Vitamin B-12, dehydrated molasses (rich in iron), bone marrow and chlorophyll. Sorry, I cannot give you the trade name, but as a clue, it is put out in tablet form by a well-known firm specializing in natural supplements, and is available at health stores.

Another vitamin deficiency leading to extreme fatigue is the lack of pantothenic acid, a B vitamin. The reason: pantothenic acid deficiency is associated with exhaustion of the adrenal glands. Tests have shown that when pantothenic acid is supplied in abundant amounts, symptoms can be relieved within three weeks.[7] Remember, though, that if you take one B vitamin alone, you must add the entire B complex, (or family) to avoid an imbalance of some of the other B vitamins which can sometimes bring results worse than the original ailment.[7]

Intestinal parasites can cause fatigue, merely because these unwanted "critters" can rob you not only of good nourishment which you need yourself, but gorge themselves on your rich red blood. Be on the alert for, and eliminate, them.[8] I like the liquid Clay Treatment mentioned in Chapter Eleven on constipation.

If you suspect hypoglycemia, you may need the help of a specialist to determine the severity of the condition through a five-hour, seven-specimen glucose tolerance test. The disturbance can usually be kept under control by plenty of protein, fresh fruits and vegetables and abstinence from coffee and manmade carbohydrates, particularly sweets.[8]

Low blood pressure, less common than high blood pressure, can cause fatigue symptoms, particularly that hard-to-get-going feeling in the morning (this also can be due to a Vitamin B deficiency). Low blood pressure is often helped by the B vitamins, particularly pantothenic acid, Vitamin C and abundant protein, with sufficient intestinal acid to help digest the protein.[7]

Any kind of infection in the body can cause fatigue. Vitamin C comes in handy here. There may be only a temporary deficiency of the vitamin or a more serious shortage of it resulting in the ailment, scurvy, as old as the hills, but more prevalent today than you or doctors may realize.[9]

Still another common cause of fatigue is a sluggish thyroid. Thyroid deficiency often responds to a *small* addition of iodine, for which most doctors have their favorite formula. Kelp tablets also contain iodine, and brewer's yeast has been found helpful in some sluggish thyroid cases. Too much iodine can make you jittery, shaky and overstimulated, so unless you use it in food form, it is safer to lean on your doctor for correct dosage.

An unsuspected cause of fatigue is allergy, particularly to ersatz food. This is not only surprising, but is new information. Stephen D. Lockey, M.D., an allergist and Chief Emeritus, Department of Allergy, Lancaster General Hospital, Lancaster, Pennsylvania, has found hidden causes of allergy in foods and drugs. He points out that thousands of additives, including artificial flavors, colors and preservatives can cause trouble. He suspects dairy products from cows treated with penicillin (to which some people are violently allergic). He has found that artificial color is found even in some synthetic multivitamin combinations, as well as in gelatin desserts, frozen desserts, candies, carbonated beverages, bakery products, cereals, even chewing gum.

He has discovered unlimited chemicals in unlimited foods, beverages, cosmetics which have caused everything from hives and headaches to gastrointestinal distress. In one case he found that sudden weakness and extreme fatigue in a physician's own family was traced to cereals and instant potatoes, both fortified with the preservatives BHA and BHT.[10]

For protection against such insidious chemicals hidden in food beverages and other products, *read your labels*. For example, we have been brainwashed long enough that BHA and BHT "won't hurt you," when actually they are potentially dangerous. Try to find a cereal or dry product on supermarket shelves without it!

What Minerals Help?

Potassium is a must to protect against fatigue. Adelle Davis reported a study done with healthy volunteers who were given refined foods for one week. These foods were the kind most Americans eat daily. Among other symptoms, the volunteers developed extreme fatigue, which disappeared almost immediately when 10 grams of potassium chloride was given them.[7] Raw, green vegetables are rich in potassium. So keep up your salads.

Calcium, another mineral which is a relaxer, may be needed for insomnia, or tension, both of which can lead to fatigue. Vitamin D (from sensibly timed sun exposure or cod liver oil) is also needed to help the calcium become absorbed by the body.

You may be startled to hear that a lack of sodium can cause fatigue, until you remember that in heat prostration sodium is urged immediately. If you have a tired, draggy feeling, you may suspect sodium deficiency. A salt deficiency can be dangerous, in spite of all the urgings shouted aloft about low-salt or salt-free diets. On the contrary, many doctors have found that at least 500 mg. of salt should be taken daily. It is true that sea salt, which contains sodium, as well as all other trace minerals, is preferable to sodium chloride, which appears in most table salt shakers and is probably responsible for adverse effects. One doctor urges his patients to eat salty foods when they feel "washed out" especially in hot weather, and another doctor gives his heart patients sea salt dissolved in water to sip to prevent heart attacks or to help control abnormal heart symptoms.[8]

Zinc deficiency is also involved in fatigue. Henry A. Schroeder, M.D., a trace mineral expert, believes that at least 10 mg. of zinc are needed daily.[11]

If there is no specific deficiency of minerals, it is wise to take a natural source of them all in kelp, natural sea salt or in filtered uncontaminated sea water (at all health stores). Minerals in homeopathic form also are found in the Schuessler Cell Salts.

A Common Cause of Fatigue

One of the most common, unsuspected causes of fatigue is

due to poisons and toxins resulting from air, soil and water pollution. Insecticides have long taken their toll, but are usually hushed up so that the insecticide industry will not be blamed. Radioactive fallout is another insidious cause, and is also pooh-poohed by those who are trying to hide the truth from the public, but which I have revealed in my book, *Are You Radioactive? How to Protect Yourself.* Radiation lodging in the body can make you bone-weary, which no amount of rest can cure. (Remedies appear in the book).[12]

Algin has been found by McGill University to protect against or neutralize radiation in the body. Look for such products as sodium alginate or magnesium alginate, etc., at health stores. *Alginate* is the clue to watch for. It comes from algin, a derivative of sea kelp.

Other toxins in the body can be eliminated by the liquid clay method, described in the chapter on constipation, or by an occasional brief fruit or juice fast to cleanse the body as a whole.

Another unexpected cause of fatigue results from the heavy toxic metals such as lead, mercury, cadmium and copper. Fluorides, too, can cause extreme fatigue. Robert Fand, M.D., states that drinking a glass of fluoridated water produces an almost instant muscle weakness which can be tested by any examiner.[13]

The other heavy metal toxins are equally disturbing. As I stated in my book, *Know Your Nutrition,* one woman had been suffering from unexplained depression and fatigue that no doctor could pinpoint because of the similarity to symptoms of many other causes. Finally, one of the growing number of alert physicians sent a sample of her hair to a testing laboratory, where it was discovered that she was loaded with lead. On questioning her, the doctor found that she had been accustomed to drinking coffee from a silver-lead cup.

But lead poisoning can come from other sources: car and plane exhaust, soil (through foods raised on it), water and air. I have related elsewhere how Dr. Harvey Ashmead took 1,000 samples of soil, water, even snow, on an automobile trip from

Salt Lake City to Chicago and, on testing, found lead in every single sample!

There *are* antidotes for heavy metal poisoning. Vitamin C can help neutralize lead and cadmium poisoning, and certain homeopathic substances can take care of the rest. (These remedies are listed in *Know Your Nutrition*.)[6] Zinc is an important antidote for lead and cadmium, but soy protein is an antagonist to zinc.

Yet, in spite of this bewildering array of disturbing factors in our environment today, probably the worst in history, there is a way out. A strong body and mind can resist the deluge of disturbers, whereas a weak mind and body cannot. A body can be built up by optimum nutrition so that all glands and organs give not only top performance but provide resistance against attack from outside elements as well. Believe it or not, constructive thinking can also be a protection, as I have described in my somewhat unusual book, *Help Yourself to Health*.[14]

Life is not easy these days. If you want something important, you must work at it, not give up easily. The rewards are well worth the effort, even may lead to the survival of the fittest, as in overcoming fatigue which many people are giving in to unnecessarily.

So search for the causes of your fatigue and outwit it before it outwits you. Check the following summary of the causes of fatigue I have listed, then work at correcting them:

1. Unresolved emotional problems or being compulsive.
2. Poor circulation.
3. Poor quality non-nutritious food.
4. Leaning on artificial "crutches": aspirin, pep pills, tranquilizers and other drugs, unlimited coffee, sweets, alcohol.
5. Lack of protein and fat, liver, brewer's yeast.
6. Eating three "squares" daily.
7. Vitamin deficiencies:
    vitamin B complex
    pantothenic acid
    folic acid and B-12 (both B vitamins)

vitamin C
vitamin D
vitamin E

8. Ailments:
   hypoglycemia
   infection
   parasites
   anemia
   low blood pressure
   allergy

9. Mineral deficiencies:
   iron
   potassium
   calcium
   sodium
   zinc

10. Lack of Hydrochloric acid for digestion.

11. Pollutants and Toxins:
    insecticides
    heavy metals: lead, mercury, cadmium, copper.
    radiation
    fluorides

REFERENCES
(See *Bibliography* for fuller details.)

1. E. Cheraskin, M.D., D.M.D., and W. M. Ringsdorf, Jr., D.M.D., M.S., *New Hope for Incurable Diseases.*

2. U.S. Department of Agriculture, Agricultural Research Service, *Food Consumption of Households in the United States.* Spring, 1965. Household Food Consumption Survey, Reports 1–5, 1968, Washington D.C., U.S. Government Printing Office.

3. Adelle Davis, *Let's Eat Right to Keep Fit.*

4. Linda Clark, *Stay Young Longer*, p. 179.

5. *Ibid*, p. 184.

6. Linda Clark, *Know Your Nutrition.*

7. Adelle Davis, *Let's Get Well*.
8. Alan H. Nittler, M.D., *A New Breed of Doctor*. (See also: Linda Clark, *Get Well Naturally*, chapter on intestinal parasites.)
9. Irwin Stone, *Vitamin C Against Disease*.
10. *Consumer's Research*, May, 1974.
11. Henry A. Schroeder, M.D., *The Trace Elements and Man*.
12. Linda Clark, *Are You Radioactive? How to Protect Yourself*.
13. *National Fluoridation News*, Oct.–Dec., 1973.
14. Linda Clark, *Help Yourself to Health*.

16: HEADACHES

(Including Migraine)

There are a host of different varieties of headaches, with as many remedies to treat them. Don't make the mistake of thinking that one remedy is the answer to them all. Taking an aspirin or gulping down a tranquilizer gives temporary relief, yes, but merely masks the condition. It does not remove the cause, which may reappear again and again until you find the correct treatment to *prevent* that type of headache.

Types of Headaches

To give you some idea of the assortment of types of headaches, here are the usual, common species. (Suggested natural, drugless treatment will follow for each.)

Allergy
Emotions
Eyestrain
High blood pressure

Hangover
Infections
Low Blood Sugar
Migraine
Nutritional deficiency
Poisons, Toxins, Smog, Radiation
Sinus
Stomach—Indigestion
Stress—Tension

In an interview with Arnold P. Friedman, M.D., Physician-in-Chief of the Montefiore Hospital Headache Unit, New York City, as well as Chairman of the World Commission for the study of Headache, Jane E. Brody, of *The New York Times,* reported, "Every day, whether watching television, listening to the radio, reading newspapers or magazines or riding in buses or trains, the sufferer—and nonsufferer—is deluged with advertising advice on the fastest, surest, safest way to get rid of headaches. More than 200 analgesic tablets to relieve headaches are on the market.

"Their basic ingredient is aspirin—acetylsalicylic acid. But they may also contain caffeine, antacids, extra pain killers, antihistamines, vitamins or mild tanquilizers.

"Dr. Friedman believes that many people take too much aspirin and related drugs, thereby masking the symptom—a headache—with pain killers instead of getting at the real trouble.

"He points out that most people do not seek medical help until over-the-counter headache preparations fail to relieve their suffering. Then they may spend years searching for a doctor who is able to help them."[1]

It is possible that you will need the help of a doctor if you cannot locate the cause of your headache. But before doing so, check the previous list to see if you can identify the cause of your headache and choose the appropriate remedies, which follow, to solve your own problem. You may, by this method, be able to obtain relief and prevent recurrence as well as save the time of the busy doctor.

Allergy

Allergy is an often overlooked cause of headache. Since allergies vary in different individuals, what will cause a headache in one, may not in another. Allergy headache may or may not be accompanied by stuffy, runny nose, often resulting from such foods as milk or milk products. Sneezing, and diarrhea are further clues to allergy, so watch for such signals which may accompany your headache.

Dr. Friedman says, "There is nearly always more to a headache than just a pain in the head." As an example, Dr. Friedman tells of a man who had headaches that recurred only on Thanksgiving and Christmas. There were three common factors on these headache days: he always ate and drank a lot; his mother-in-law always came for dinner, and the main dish was always turkey. It took several years to pinpoint the cause. Each year the turkeys were ordered from the same farm where they had been fed mash later found to contain penicillin. As it turned out, the man was allergic to penicillin!

For more suggestions see Chapter Three on Allergies.

Emotions

Entire books have been written on the effects of emotions, so I will merely remind you that headaches can be caused by intense emotions. You have no doubt heard the saying that one can be "allergic" to another person. Even husbands and wives can be allergic to each other, or to mothers-in-law who are the "pain-in-the-neck" type. Adelle Davis also noted that "Migraine headaches are often caused by early anger and frequently disappear during psychotherapy."[2]

Many people who appear to have a sweet disposition, may actually be sizzling inside about a condition, a job, resentment toward a boss, or some other hostility which they keep buried from the public (even themselves) but which manifest as headaches. Negative feelings should not be bottled up, but expressed in some safe way. If it is not possible to "ventilate" to the person who irritates you, then psychotherapy or a constructive outlet for the hostility should be found before you blow a fuse.

I once knew a man who hated his job with a vengeance, yet he was stuck with it. At that time there was no other job available to support him and his family, so he chose a wise substitute for blowing off steam to prevent the pressure headaches that were plaguing him. Every night, after dinner, he would take refuge in his woodworking shop in the basement and hammer the day-lights out of the wood which he eventually turned into some beautiful pieces of furniture.

Adelle Davis used to tell those who were ready to blow to get a pillow, give it the name of the person or problem bugging them, and either beat the pillow to smithereens or put it on the floor and kick it violently every time they passed it.

When pressure is released harmlessly, it usually does not cause an emotional pressure headache.

Emotions are tricky; they can hide from their owner, who is often the last to see and admit the cause. Usually one is too hasty in blaming the other fellow. So if self-searching does not bring the real problem to light, get help from a counselor: a psychologist, psychiatrist, minister, or understanding friend.

Eyestrain

A common source of headaches. See your oculist, or do eye exercises, or both.

High Blood Pressure Headaches

Those who suffer from high blood pressure are rarely in doubt as to the cause of their pounding or constricting headaches. There is a safe method of treatment available now. Charlotte Yale, a nutritionist who counsels patients under the aegis of physicians, psychiatrists and psychologists, reports a technique she learned in Europe: Sit on the edge of a bathtub which contains water as hot as you can stand, immerse your legs up to the calves only for fifteen to twenty minutes. This draws the blood away from the head and down to the feet, bringing relief from the headache.

Hangover

There are those who claim that alcohol constricts the blood vessels. Others believe it causes the blood vessels to swell, resulting in that painful morning-after headache. I hesitate to give you the following remedy because it would be better in the long run for you to avoid alcohol in large amounts and thus decline to become an alcoholic. There are already too many alcoholics. (See Chapter Two on Alcoholism.)

However, here is the remedy. I hope you will not abuse or overdo it. The Navy, I am told, discovered during World War II that if you took one Vitamin B-1 (thiamin) tablet with your drink (no more potent than 5 or 10 mg. each), you would avoid a hangover headache. Vitamin B-1 is just dandy, but many of you know by now that if you take too much of one of the B factors, without the addition of the entire B family, known as the B complex, you are in for trouble. The overuse of one factor, particularly B-1, can cause imbalance of the other B factors in your body and cause troubles you could do without. (This is explained in my book, *Know Your Nutrition*, available at book and health stores).[3]

You will receive some protection from this imbalance if you will take, in addition to the B-1, the whole B complex in liberal amounts *the same day,* preferably in the form of wheat germ, brewer's yeast or liver. The latter can be fresh or desiccated, in tablet form. All these foods are among the richest sources of the B complex.

The reason for the use of the Vitamin B-1 with alcohol is that alcohol steals it from your body, playing havoc with your nerves, which the B-1 is supposed to protect.

Infections

If you will stop to think about it, a headache is a common occurrence when you have an infection. It is often present when you have a cold, a virus, a fever, or whatever. So it may be a clue to the fact that you are developing something. Or it may be the result of an infection already in full bloom. In any case, the sensible approach is to attack not the headache, but the infection. The best all-round method I know of to accomplish this is to load up on Vitamin C. If a cold is coming on, as I have always said and will continue to say, start the Vitamin C therapy the *minute* the first symptom shows up. I have heard people claim that Vitamin C cures a cold. Not so in my family. It may lighten or shorten it somewhat, but it won't stop it in its tracks once the cold has taken hold. But if you do not delay a minute when you notice the first symptoms that herald a cold for you: scratchy throat, runny nose, etc., and keep after it with massive doses every hour, Vitamin C has worked miracles. At the first symptom, all of my family and friends and nutritionally oriented specialists, take 1,000 mg. of ascorbic acid every hour, plus a calcium tablet to buffer it and prevent nervousness. (This has long been recommended by both Adelle Davis and Fred R. Klenner, M.D., who has done extensive research with Vitamin C on his patients.)

If you want a postage stamp coverage of the many other infections Vitamin C can help, see my book, *Know your Nutrition*.[3] You will find still more in the book by Irwin Stone.[4] Researchers who have worked with Vitamin C for years, state that those scare stories about this vitamin may be an attempt to brainwash the public, since they simply are not true, according to their findings supported by laboratory studies.

So if you are a victim of an infection, get to work with Vitamin C. It may be safer than an antibiotic; in fact it is considered a *natural* antibiotic. If your infection is a life-and-death matter, then your doctor will have to decide which to take. Once you have controlled the infection with massive doses of Vitamin C, you will probably begin to taper off with doses every few hours, then every few days until you are free from discomfort as well as the headache which may have accompanied the infection.

Remember that a headache is nature's way of telling you that something is amiss in your body. Better listen and use a natural remedy instead of questionable medicines which have, for some people, actually caused headaches. I have seen it happen.

Low Blood Sugar (Hypoghycemia)

Low blood sugar is one of the most common, yet unsuspected, causes of irritability and headache. That all-gone feeling before meals, or the four o'clock slump, is often accompanied by headache. Briefly, such things as too much coffee, too infrequent meals, too many carbohydrates—most hypoglycemics crave sweets, thus compounding the problem—may lead to this ailment, widely common today. A missed breakfast, a hurried sandwich-and-dessert lunch, all laced with numerous coffee breaks, can lead you straight into low blood sugar which often brings on headaches. I will repeat for the rare person who still thinks that sugar is the cure of low blood sugar: *It is not.* It raises the blood sugar temporarily, and makes you feel better for a little while, but is soon followed by a nosedive of blood sugar during which time you feel shaky, irritable, headachy, and like snarling at your best friends. You may even black out. Many accidents have been caused by low blood sugar. And those parents who lecture their children and husbands not to eat between meals should, in my opinion, be restrained. I have stated elsewhere that when family members become irritable just before meals—a sign of low blood sugar—I rush a snack to them if a full meal is not ready, and suddenly everyone is cheerful and happy once more. If a headache has already developed, it is probably on its way out. Low blood sugar may be the cause of your husband coming home and grabbing a cocktail until dinner is ready. He is unknowingly reaching for a life line to raise his blood sugar.

Low blood sugar is not a figment of the imagination; it is the result of an abused pancreas which overstimulates the production of insulin in the body. Yet it is surprisingly simple to control: eat smaller meals more often, rather than forcing yourself to wait for three large "squares" daily; cut manmade carbohydrates to the bone; substitute protein, and eliminate coffee, one of the greatest causes of low blood sugar because it overstimulates the pancreas, particularly when no protein food is taken with it. This program has brought remarkable results and a feeling of well-being, as well as prevented low blood sugar headache.

Adelle Davis stated, "Low blood sugar is another frequent

cause of migraine headaches. In thirty-five migraine sufferers, studied by electroencephalograms for five hours during severe headaches, all had low blood sugar. The lower the blood sugar, the more severe the headaches."[2]

But there is more to the story of migraine headaches as you will see in what follows.

Migraine Headaches

Many doctors insist that there is no cure for migraine headache except drugs which, they admit, merely bring temporary relief, or an operation. I disagree. I speak from experience since I was, at one time, a migraine sufferer, and licked the problem without drugs. I have told my story in my book, *Get Well Naturally*, but I have learned even more about those excruciating headaches since I wrote that book. They *are* preventable, and I have proved it to my own—and others'—satisfaction.

Migraine headaches (sometimes called sick headaches) can be due to an allergy, or a migraine personality.[5] I plead guilty to both. As a child I was given chocolate to eat or drink, and it took many years before I saw the connection between the chocolate (a common allergen for many unsuspecting persons) and what was at that time called "bilious" headaches. Once when I talked with a doctor, I mentioned this fact, and he said, "Well, if I knew of something that was upsetting me I would give it up—and quick." I did, though I still love chocolate. Fortunately I can substitute carob, which is more nutritious, available in health stores, and tastes almost the same. But that was not the end of my migraines. Meanwhile I had, for other reasons, apparently developed a migraine personality, as I explained in *Get Well Naturally*.

Other foods to which some people are allergic and which can trigger migraine headaches, according to Dr. Donald Dalessio, Professor of Neurology at the University of Kentucky, are chicken livers, pickled herring, alcohol, some wines, strong cheese, canned figs, monosodiumglutamate, and cured meats including ham, bacon, hot dogs, salami, etc. (All of these cured meats contain the disturbing nitrates and nitrites.)

People with migraine personalities are compulsive workers as well as perfectionists, feel that they have to do everything *now*, and will usually tell you, "I will rest when I have finished my chores." When they do finish, they let down suddenly from a state of temporary but great tension, to a luxurious feeling of relief that their work is over. Bingo, comes the migraine! It is purely a physiological process. Dr. Arnold Friedman, the headache expert mentioned earlier, explains that the head and neck muscles, reacting from continuous stress, can become overworked just as an overworked arm muscle. The tight muscle can squeeze arteries and reduce blood flow. Then when the person *lets down suddenly, and all the way* (the clue to maigraine), the constricted muscles expand, stretching the blood vessel walls. Each time the sufferer's heart beats, the blood being pushed through these vessels expands them further and causes the excruciating pain.

Thanks to research work from two doctors, Thomas Holmes, M.D., University of Washington Medical School, and the late Sol Hirsch, M.D., of New York City, I finally learned what to do to prevent these headaches. Dr. Holmes cautioned, "If you have tightened up to meet a deadline (self-imposed, usually) don't let down all at once, but little by little so that the blood flow can be held in check and the blood vessels relax gradually, not suddenly. Intersperse work with rest; work a while, rest a while, by degrees. Dr. Hirsch agreed that a work schedule should be balanced with rest, work and play which does not permit you to get too tense or overworked in the first place. If you don't allow yourself to get too steamed up, it is easier to get back to normal. I had to teach myself a mañana or "so-what" attitude. If I didn't get everything I wanted to do done today, I decided, so what? I can finish tomorrow. I finally re-educated myself and I almost never have a migraine headache anymore.

The doctor of a friend of mine who is migraine-prone told her that the appearance of the migraine is a signal to unschedule herself.

Dr. Holmes, however, gave tips about what to do if a migraine has already started. Migraine headaches always give fair warning. The victim will see flashes of light, or only parts of objects in front of him. He may also feel a tingling, numbness, or weakness in an arm or leg. This does not last long, disappearing as the headache takes over and pain commences. If this happens, says Dr. Holmes, *do not give in to it.* Never go to bed in a darkened room and warn everyone to go away. If you do, you will probably be there for three days (the usual life of a migraine) with violent nausea, vomiting and incredible, continuous pain. Instead, stay on your feet in the daytime. Do simple chores which do not require too much concentration. Walk, move around, get some fresh air, and drink some coffee! Coffee seems to be an antidote and cuts down on blood vessel expansion. It "tightens" them up a bit. If you want to sleep at night, *Anacin* and other painkillers that contain caffeine seem to work better than those without caffeine. But another doctor has a still better suggestion which I have also tried and passed on to many others, with great success.

The remedy is niacin (formerly called nicotinic acid), a B vitamin. When you take it, there is usually an intense flush which gradually spreads over your entire body and lasts about fifteen minutes. You may turn beet red, and burn or ·itch, but it is definitely harmless if used in the proper dosage recommended by doctors. The discomfort is a drop in the bucket compared to the torturous migraine. Lewis J. Silvers, M.D., says, "At the very first symptoms, even if they awaken you out of a deep sleep, immediately take a 50 mg. tablet of niacin (at drug or health stores). If a flush ensues, the dose is sufficient to quickly dilate the constricted cerebral blood vessels. If you do not get a flush in ten minutes, take another tablet to produce a flush. Presto—no migraine!"[6]

Still more help comes from homeopathy. A. Dwight Smith, M.D., a homeopathic physician tells of curing his mother who had suffered from migraines for twenty-five years. When she was fifty-five, Dr. Smith had just finished his training in homeopathy. His mother woke up one morning with a migraine and he gave her a homeopathic powder known as *Pulsatilla* 10M (available from homeopathic physicians only). He returned home expecting his mother to be in bed in terrible agony and retching as usual. To his surprise she was up and working. She said her headache was practically gone by the time she took the second powder. She lived twenty-nine years longer and never had another migraine, he reports. Dr. Smith warns that not all homeopathic remedies fit all people. It is necessary for the homeopathic doctor to use the remedy to fit the individual, which may take a varying length of time.[7](Also see this reference to find out where a homeopathic physician is in your area.)

However, I discovered a homeopathic substance mentioned in *Get Well Naturally* that anyone can buy at a homeopathic pharmacy. It has worked for many. It is called *Iris Ver.* 6X. After reading the chapter on migraine in that book and taking the *Iris* 6X, a reader wrote me, "*Iris* 6X is nothing if not magic. I had suffered from migraines for fifteen to twenty years, been to neurologists, psychiatrists and other specialists. I had even been hospitalized with medication, tests and under observation. All this did for me was to considerably deplete my bank account. The migraines persisted. I have taken no more than 10 *Iris* 6X in the past ten years (they are the size of the head of a pin) and *no more migraines!*"

There is one strange thing about migraines that no one has been able to explain. Dr. Sol Hirsch noted it, and most migraine sufferers, once their attention is called to it, will agree. After the migraine has been routed, the person feels a brief rebound of energy. Dr. Hirsch stated that it was his belief that migraine steps in in the midst of great tension and stress and may be likened to the popping of a safety valve. "Once it is over," he said, "it is my belief that the migraine attack has restored energy to the body to balance the stress it has experienced."[5]

Dr. Hirsch also found that nutritional deficiency plays a part in headaches. Adelle Davis, as you would expect, agreed. Let's look at that type of headache next.

Nutritional Deficiency Headaches

A lack of iron, resulting in anemia, is a common cause of headache. The headache sometimes appears before the anemia, due to a chronic iron shortage. Not all types of iron are considered safe or acceptable by nutritionists and doctors. This applies to foods fortified with iron (see Chapter 4). However, Adelle Davis has written, "Brewers or nutritional yeast is such an excellent source of iron that anemia can easily be prevented by taking a few teaspoons daily."[2] But headaches can also result from the deficiency of B vitamins, namely pantothenic acid, B-1 (thiamin), B-12 and B-6 (pyridoxine).[8]

Allergy headaches are often helped by taking pantothenic acid, a B vitamin. Do not look for overnight relief here, since pantothenic acid helps to repair damaged adrenal glands, the protective watchdogs of the body. This takes several weeks after the diet is improved.[2] Adelle Davis reported the case of a physician who suffered severe reactions from pollen and house dust who noticed relief soon after beginning pantothenic acid. But he found that he could remain symptom-free only as long as he continued the pantothenic acid.[2]

Both Vitamins B-1 and B-12 have also helped headaches, including migraines.[2]

B-6 deficiency is attracting more and more attention, since apparently it has a finger in so many pies. John M. Ellis, M.D. points out, as a result of his many years' work with B-6 on thousands of patients, that a lack of it contributes to brain hyperirritability as well as edema (a swelling of body tissues) which could lead to headache. He cites one case of headache in a woman in her fourth month of pregnancy. The headache had persisted for two weeks. Dr. Ellis usually administers B-6 (also known as pyridoxine) in doses ranging from 50 to 100 mg. daily, but in this case increased the dosage to 225 milligrams daily. The headaches stopped! Apparently the added stress of pregnancy required more B-6.[8]

Again let me caution you, when taking any of the separate B vitamin factors, to add to your diet *the same day* the entire B complex in some form: brewer's yeast, liver, wheat germ, etc. Otherwise too much of one factor can throw the other factors into imbalance causing other undesirable problems.[8] Actually, the entire B complex itself is a protector against headaches, including migraine. The late Sol Hirsch, M.D., prescribed large amounts of desiccated whole liver daily (usually up to 18 capsules of 0.5 grams each) for a feeling of well-being, body repair and defense against headaches.[5]

The late D. C. Jarvis, M.D., in his book on Vermont Folk Medicine,[10] used still another remedy for chronic headaches. He noted that although headaches are usually blamed on eyes, stomach, kidneys, liver, sinuses and emotions, all of which can be true, his approach was to restore natural acidity to the body in order to combat overalkalinity, this despite the many commercials urging antacids. Since the symptoms of too much acid and too much alkalinity are identical (except in cases of ulcer where acid should be withheld), most people are confused into thinking that acid is a dirty word. Not true. If one does not have sufficient natural acid in the body, protein, iron and calcium cannot be digested.[9]

Dr. Jarvis found that taking a little apple cider vinegar in water daily, or two teaspoons of honey, or both, will stop a headache, even a migraine, within one half hour. He says it will also disappear in one half hour if you will place equal parts of apple cider vinegar in water in a steamer, cover your head with a towel and inhale 75 breaths. Apple cider vinegar also contains minerals which most people need.[10]

Poisons, Toxins, Smog, Radiation

Poisons and toxins admitted into the body through food, beverages, and water, as well as through breathing today's air, can undoubtedly cause a myriad of disturbances. A headache may be the first warning that a poison has entered your body. Additives in foods are serious offenders, and in many cases, including cosmetics, skin and hair products, the ingredients are not listed on the label, thus producing a hazard for some people who are not even aware of it. Witness the example of the man (described under allergies) who developed headaches from eating penicillin-fed turkey. It took several years of detective work to pinpoint that cause. Some causes are never found.

Cleaning products in the home, school or office can be breathed, resulting in headaches too. Since up to 10,000 chemicals, including pesticides, colorings, flavorings, preservatives, propellant gas in spray cans, plus countless others, are allowed, or placed deliberately in the products we eat, drink and use, no wonder the body can react to a poison with a headache as a result of an offending foreign substance that has invaded it.

In addition, toxic air contaminants are also too numerous to mention. Smog alone contains many chemicals belched forth from car exhausts, which are rightly given the greatest blame, and from industrial chimneys, which provide us with fluorides, the heavy toxic metals such as lead, mercury, and cadmium, sulphuric acid, and asbestos, plus hundreds—perhaps thousands—of other contaminants. Of all of these, radiation is the most dangerous. You can't see it, you can't feel it, but it is deadly just the same.

Nuclear bombs and plants are not only lethal, but so are other manmade devices. I recently learned of a woman who had had periodic headaches for six years. They were finally traced to radiation from fluorescent lights in her office, and to anemia.[11]

Another woman told me that she suffered from eye-aches as well as headaches in college classrooms equipped with fluorescent lights. she finally began to wear a hat to class, thereby provoking laughter from the other students. She said, "I would rather be laughed at than suffer from headaches, which ceased when I started wearing the hat for protection."

Radiation is said by researchers at McGill University in Canada to be neutralized in the body by algin, a derivative of kelp. This appears in various products at health stores, such as magnesium alginate, sodium alginate, etc. Cadmium is also said to respond to the alginates. There is also help for lead and mercury poisoning.

The most recent method of detecting lead poisoning is by hair analysis from a few laboratories. Your doctor can take a hair sample and send it in for analysis. (The laboratories do not deal with patients, only doctors.) In addition to the alginates (available at health stores in powder or tablet form), Vitamin C has been found to help victims of lead poisoning. But there are two other simple methods you can use at home, as suggested by John J. Miller, Ph.D., as follows:

For lead poisoning, use from ¼ to ½ cup of baked beans daily. The sulfhydryl substance in vegetable baked beans helps chelate the lead for its removal from the body. Dr. Miller has isolated this chelating agent from the baked beans and makes it available in a product called *Ledex* (available through doctors and pharmacies, from Miller Pharmacal Co., Box 299, West Chicago, Illinois 60185). A laboratory associated with this company also does the hair analysis. *Ledex* can be used by anyone except those with low calcium.

Dr. Miller has a simple home remedy for mercury, too. It is applesauce, which neutralizes the mercury. Make your own applesauce. Omit the stem and the bottom area. Cut the rest of the apple into small pieces. Cook over low heat without sugar.

What else can you do to protect yourself?

-For more radiation protections, see my book, *Are You Radioactive? How to Protect Yourself*. (Available through book and health stores.[11])

-Read your labels on foods and beverages and reject those with chemicals, even though you do not understand the terms. As I have so often said, if you can't pronounce the name of an additive, don't buy the product.

-Raise what food you can and buy, if possible, organic food, uncontaminated with pesticides. After recently witnessing strawberries in commercial fields being doused with arsenic, and spinach and artichokes being sprayed with DDT and other pesticides from planes, I refuse to buy such commercial products at all.

The best preventive remedy I know is to build up your body resistance through superhealth by nutrition, exercise and constructive thinking.

For further nutritional fortification, please read my book *Know Your Nutrition*[3] (available in paperback at health and book stores.)

Sinus

Sinus headaches plague many people. A nutritional suggestion is the use of Vitamin A in sensible amounts. If you do not take it in capsule form, it is available in cod liver oil (I use the mint-flavored, and mix it ice cold with fruit juice, taking one tablespoon daily from a separate little jar reserved for it only). Vitamin A, especially as found in cod liver oil, is healing to mucous membranes.

The home remedies may help when all else fails. If the sinus headache has already made its appearance, placing hot, wet towels across the sinus area for a while every day for three days, helps to relieve the congestion causing the headache. But you can help *prevent* sinus complaints by another remedy which is close to magical in its effect: chlorophyll. By diluting the water-soluble type so it won't sting on contact, or using the oil-soluble type, which does not smart (both in liquid form at health stores), and transferring it to a sterile dropper bottle purchased from a drugstore, you can put a drop or so in each nostril every night at bedtime, as well as in the morning. It has worked wonders for many grateful sinus sufferers. Taking large amounts of Vitamin C can also help.

Stomach—Indigestion Headaches

Who hasn't had a stomach headache? Indiscriminate eating, drinking, air or car sickness, sometimes intensified by heat and other factors, can cause headaches. See Chapter 17 on Indigestion for suggestions. Apple cider vinegar or hydrochloric acid may bring great relief.

Stress—Tension Headaches

Stress and tension headaches are probably the most common of all, particularly for sedentary workers. Since such headaches have similar causes as "sick headaches," see Migraine Headaches for suggestions on how to avoid them. Otherwise try to relieve the stress that produced the headache in the first place.

Take some time at your desk, *before* the headache develops, by doing the well-known head and neck exercises. This is merely rotating your head, with fully stretched neck, frontward and backward three times each, and then three times clockwise to the right, and three times counterclockwise to the left. Many report eye tension also disappears with these exercises. Car drivers during long trips should stop and do these exercises, too.

For all-over body tension from pushing yourself too hard, often a factor in headache, get up out of your chair, walk around, stretch, and breathe deeply. If you already have a headache, it may disappear as your circulation is restored. If you can relax before the headache appears, you can help prevent its onset.

If your neck tension is chronic, see your chiropractor or osteopath. Perhaps your atlas-axis area is out of alignment, cutting off the circulation to your head, resulting in the headache. It takes only a few minutes to have this adjustment and is well worth it.

To Use or Not to Use?

Should you avoid using painkillers? My answer may surprise some of you.

It is true that aspirin has a lot against it, but usually this is because so many people take too many aspirin daily. If you take one to stop excruciating pain, say, once every six months or a year, this is not going to do you in, particularly if you later take some Vitamin C to neutralize its effect. Pain, in itself, can cause stress, and you will have to decide which is worse—the stress or the pain. You may well opt for temporary help from a painkiller. Meanwhile you can work on the basic cause of your headache, which may take longer.

One more thing: there are different types of over-the-counter painkillers. Some have salicylic acid, to which many people are extremely allergic. If you belong to this class, there is a new type which contains *acetaminophen* instead of *acetylsalicylic* acid and has a good record for safety. Two brands containing *acetaminophen* available at drugstores are *Tylenol* and *Nebs*. Another, *C-Ophen*, is available at some health stores, in time-released tablets also containing Vitamin C, zinc, potassium and magnesium to help the body combat stress as well as pain. It is manufactured by the Alacer Corporation, Box 6166 Buena Park, California, 90622.

I must warn you, though, that if you are trying to subdue a migraine which got away from you, I have found that only the painkiller with caffeine in it does the job.

So let your conscience be your guide. Don't become a slave to painkillers. Instead, outwit your headache intelligently.

REFERENCES
(See *Bibliography* for fuller details.)

1. *The New York Times*, March 4, 1968.
2. Adelle Davis, *Let's Get Well*.
3. Linda Clark, *Know Your Nutrition*.
4. Irwin Stone, *The Healing Factor: Vitamin C Against Disease*.
5. Sol Hirsch, M.D., "Clinical Observations on Migraine and Its Treatment," *New York State Journal of Medicine*, Vol. 54, No. 5.
6. Lewis J. Silvers' *Extraordinary Remedies and Prescriptions for Health and Longevity*.
7. *Homeopathic Bulletin*, January, 1974.
8. John M. Ellis, M.D., with James Presley, *Vitamin B: The Doctor's Report*.
9. Linda Clark, *Secrets of Health and Beauty*.
10. D. C. Jarvis, M.D., *Folk Medicine*.
11. Linda Clark, *Are You Radioactive? How to Protect Yourself*.

17: INDIGESTION

Indigestion is a common ailment these days and TV commercials are not helping the situation by recommending many foods that can make the condition worse. Actually, there are an enormous number of people suffering from indigestion, some of whom do not even know it. Of course they realize something is wrong, but can't put their finger on the cause. Others who are well aware of their ailment don't know what to do about it and usually do the wrong thing. In most cases, you will find that nobody can cure your indigestion except you, yourself. This is probably because you are the one who caused it in the first place, and you must be the one to prevent it in the future.

Someone once wrote me, "I feel fine as long as I don't eat." Silly as it may sound, it may be tragically true of many indigestion sufferers. Yet we must eat to keep our body machine in good working order. So the real dilemima is *what* should we eat, and *how* should we eat it, in order to digest it properly, enabling it to nourish and strengthen our bodies and make us feel good at the same time?

What Kind of Foods Should You Eat?

Food allergies are common. You will hear people say, "Oh, I can't eat cucumbers," or cabbage, onions, strawberries, chocolate, oranges and many more. These may be true allergies for certain people (see Chapter Three). But there are other pitfalls in foods. Most foods found in regular food shopping centers today are filled or treated with numerous additives which can often be classified as poisons. The names are not always listed on the labels, and even if they were, the consumer might not understand their hazards, since the truth is purposely kept from the public by food industries to encourage more sales. The most dramatic explanation of this problem I have found is the book, *Eating May be Hazardous to Your Health*, by Jaqueline Verrett, Ph.D., with Jean Carper (Simon and Schuster, 1974). Dr. Verrett had been a biochemist and researcher for the FDA for fifteen years and not only knows firsthand what goes on behind the scenes in the FDA, but is not afraid to tell the truth of what is allowed in the foods you buy and eat. No wonder there is so much indigestion and other illness in this country! You will be doing yourself, your family and friends a service to read and recommend this book, providing you are not afraid of shocks. It is full of them.

The best solution is to eat natural, untreated, unchemicalized, untampered-with food, organically raised, even if you have to raise it yourself. There are ways of getting such food but lazy people will not qualify; you have to work at it. I hope Dr. Verrett's book will goad you into action.

However, even in the case of some natural foods, there are people who suffer from certain disturbances—those cucumbers, for example. So, if you are convinced that a food disturbs you, don't eat it. But before you give it up, try to find out *why* you can't eat it.

Some Common Causes of Indigestion and Some Cures

Acidity: Due to the influence of TV and other commercials, the average person is convinced that he is suffering from too much stomach acid and pops into his mouth an antacid tablet at the first sign of the slightest stomach distress. This is where the trouble begins. Of course, there *are* some cases of hyperacidity, but they are the *exceptions*, not the rule. Ulcer patients, plus a few others, may belong to this group. But the average person has *too little acid* and this is the cause of his indigestion. By taking an antacid tablet he merely makes himself worse; and the more he takes the worse he gets. Why?

A healthy person manufactures an acid in his digestive tract. It is called hydrochloric acid. Formerly, as a person became older, his supply of hydrochloric (abbreviated as HCL) dwindled. No more. Because of widespread tension and stress, which can inhibit the manufacture of HCL, even some children today are suffering from deficiencies of this valuable, natural body acid. Another cause of its lack can be traced to a deficit of B vitamins. Some babies lack HCL due to poor diet or tension, or both, in their mother prior to birth, or afterwards in themselves. Reports show that some babies who were born less than healthy have been brought to better health quickly by the addition of a diluted amount of HCL to their formula.

HCL is needed to help the body digest protein, iron and calcium (the weak babies could not digest their milk, which contains both protein and calcium). Adults with insufficient HCL also do not digest meat, fowl, fish, brewers yeast, or dairy products, which produce toxins in their body from the undigested food. This is one of the major causes of the present increasing return to vegetarianism. Vegetarians claim that they feel better without protein, and they are right because they are not digesting it. So, for a while, they *do* actually feel better without the undigested food and residual toxins in their bodies. But the reckoning comes later; without adequate protein, of which the body is made, and which must be replaced regularly, the body may begin to suffer as the protein runs out. And the less protein you eat, the less HCL your body manufactures.

I wish I had kept account of the many readers who have written me telling how HCL has removed their gas (a by-product of undigested protein foods) and improved their health, after I explained the use of HCL in my book, *Secrets of Health and Beauty* (paperback at health and book stores). In that book, I reported fully the findings of Dr. E. Hugh Tuckey, one of the few doctors who has discovered the value of adding HCL to diet. I cannot repeat the whole story here, for lack of space, but I will touch on the high points.

Dr. Tuckey stated that the symptoms of too little acid are *exactly the same* as the symptoms of too much acid. Antacid tablets merely compound the problem, as does bicarbonate of soda, a common antacid. "Avoid antacids," Dr. Tuckey warned, "until you have learned if you are *really* suffering from an overacid stomach."

Dr. Tuckey's method is to use a brand of HCL which is combined with pepsin, another natural digestant found in the body. The combination is usually known as HCL Betaine-with-Pepsin. He has tried many different kinds of HCL with his patients and found this form, in tablets, the easiest to take and the most effective. (It is available in health stores.)

In order to determine whether or not HCL is for you, Dr. Tuckey (who has now retired and no longer practices) suggests taking a tablet after your main protein meal and see what happens. If all goes well, you are on the right track. But if you feel a burning sensation (very rare) then you may be one of the few who do not need it. In this case, he says, drink a whole glass of water and the acid will be washed away. Just to be sure, you might try a half tablet at another meal. Maybe you need less; you will have to experiment to find your own dosage. I know people who have been tested and have no HCL at all. I know others who have some, but not enough. Since the medical tests for a lack of HCL include stomach pumping and other less unpleasant but hard-to-find tests, Dr. Tuckey believes you can ascertain the dosage for yourself and there is no one to tell you you can't.

Dr. D. C. Jarvis, the Vermont Folk Medicine physician, suggested using another form of acid: apple cider vinegar (*no other kind*) combined with water to suit your taste, to sip with or between meals. He found this not only helped digestion, but, if taken before or immediately after eating doubtful foods which may have spoiled (such as those served at large picnics where food is held over for hours without refrigeration), and acid will neutralize the deterioration and protect you from possible food poisoning. The reason: *germs cannot survive in an acid medium.* Even Vitamin C can help here.

Intestinal Flora

There is still another method of coping with continuous, as well as temporary, digestive problems. Due to the broad use of antibiotics these days, as well as the hodge-podge of chemicals and drugs we put into our systems, to say nothing of the poor nutritional intake by the average person, our intestines can get into a sorry state so that nothing seems to agree with us. Gas, fatigue, diarrhea, constipation, heartburn (fullness, burning, sourness, pain) may result from indigestion, not in the stomach but in the intestines. For this type of indigestion, certain intestinal substances are lacking so that normal digestion cannot take place. In a healthy body, there exists a healthy intestinal "flora," which means that there are certain types of benign or "good" bacteria which work on the food to help its digestion. But antibiotics can kill these friendly bacteria and allow the unfriendly bacteria to take over. Result: incomplete digestion, often diarrhea, cramping and other problems. Flatulence (lower bowel gas) is the most common complaint. Fortunately, this is normally easy to remedy.

Poor intestinal flora can be replaced by good intestinal flora by simply taking certain foods or substances that are rich in the friendly bacteria. At first, you may experience more gas or other undesirable symptoms, due to a battle between the "good" and "bad" bacteria. But keep adding good bacteria, and the war will soon end. The good will vanquish the bad, and your innards will be left in peace. This is especially true after taking an antibiotic. European doctors know this, but for some reason many doctors in other countries haven't learned the lesson. The remedy is to take simultaneously (or close together) the soured milks such as yogurt, Kefir, or acidophilus milk, all of which contain friendly bacteria, which will go to work to propagate more of their kind and subdue the unfriendly hosts. If you need more rapid help or the problem is serious, taking acidophilus culture straight from the bottle (at health stores) will literally provide you with millions of these active, friendly bacteria at every gulp, which usually brings speedy results.

The word "gulp" gives us one more clue to establishing good digestion, plus other benefits.

Fletcherism

A woman said to me recently, "You know, I have discovered that when I gulp my food, I get indigestion. But when I chew it thoroughly, I don't." This is what Fletcherism is all about. Years ago, John D. Rockefeller put it in a nutshell. He said, "Don't gobble your food. Fletcherize, or chew slowly while you eat. Talk on pleasant topics. Don't be in a hurry. Take time to masticate and cultivate a cheerful appetite while eating, and outwit that demon, indigestion."

Fletcherism was discovered in 1898 by Horace Fletcher, M.A., a fellow of the American Association for Advancement of Science. Fletcher, at the time, was forty years old, and considered himself an "old" man. He was fifty pounds overweight, contracted flu every six months, was afflicted with a continuous "tired feeling" and was harrowed by indigestion. He applied for a life insurance policy and was turned down as a poor risk. He began to analyze his eating and experiment on himself. As he made important discoveries, he set up rules for "Fletcherism." The rules were:

1. Chew your food to a pulp or milky liquid until it practically swallows itself.

2. Never eat until hungry.

3. Enjoy every bite or morsel, savoring the flavor until it is swallowed.

4. Do not eat when tired, angry, worried, and at mealtime re-

fuse to think or talk about unpleasant subjects. (This causes tension and interferes with digestion.) He considered the most important rule of all, *complete mastication*. He tried counting at first and found that chewing less than thirty times per mouthful was insufficient. Later, chewing food to pulp or liquid became the standard.

Horace Fletcher followed these rules for five months. As a result he lost more than sixty pounds and felt better than he had for twenty years. He said, "My head was clear, my body felt springy, I enjoyed walking, and that tired feeling was gone." Two years after he began "Fletcherism," he said his strength and endurance had increased beyond his wildest expectations. On his fiftieth birthday he traveled by bicycle nearly two hundred miles over uneven French roads, and came home feeling fine with no stiffness then or afterward.

Because people would not believe his claim for endurance, he submitted himself to two universities for scientific tests. At Yale University he doubled the word's record by lifting 300 pounds of dead weight, 350 times. At the University of Pennsylvania he broke the college record for lifting power. At age sixty-four, he still maintained a normal weight, did the work of a man of forty, rarely had a cold, forgot there was such a thing as that tired feeling and slept like a baby.

Fletcher said, "I have done this simply by keeping my body free of excess food and the putrefaction of the food that the body does not want and cannot take care of."[1] The university scientists who tested Fletcher were so impressed that they, too, began to Fletcherize with similar results.

Since then, as I have written elsewhere, there is a reducing program built on Fletcherism that has worked like a charm.[2] Both Horace Fletcher and those who have tried this reducing regimen comment on their lowered food bills, an important point in these days of rising food costs. Obviously, the more nutritious the diet, the better value for the body, too.

We have long been told that thorough mastication is needed to digest starches. The reason given, is that starch or carbohydrate should be well mixed with the saliva, since its digestion begins in the mouth. But digestion of protein takes place in the stomach. This was learned from studies with dogs fed meat tied to a string which was withdrawn after swallowing. The meat had been automatically digested by the HCL without previous chewing. Today, however, with HCL shortage in people becoming more and more common, perhaps the thorough mastication of protein, too, is advisable to prepare it for a less-than-normal supply of HCL in the stomach. Thorough mastication does take more time but it also gives greater results.

Many writers on the subject of indigestion caution against negative thinking or conversation at meals. Worry, anxiety, fear, anger, hatred, resentment and apprehension can temporarily paralyze the manufacture of digestive elements, including HCL. Parents should forbid children from bickering at the table and should refrain from arguments themselves. Don't read or watch TV either. Music with your meals is all right, if you like it. Some don't. I have written before of an elderly woman with whom I lunched regularly. The minute we sat down at the table she would regale me with the illnesses and deaths of her friends, complete with all of their unpleasant symptoms. My stomach curled into a knot until I tactfully changed the subject.

Other Helps

There are some herbs, which drunk in tea form can help indigestion. Some of these are spices such as anise, allspice, cloves, and others.[3] My grandmother used to drink hot ginger tea for indigestion or "settling the stomach." Another stomach "settler" is mint tea. *Potter's Cyclopaedia*, originally published in 1907, described mint as, "Used for allaying nausea, flatulence, sickness and vomiting."[4]

In the summertime, at my house, I make mint iced tea. I raise my own mint and steep a handful of it with regular weak tea, also considered by some a stomach settler. I pour the tea warm over ice cubes, serve it chilled without sugar and guests always clamor for more.

B vitamins help digestion, especially thiamine (B-1) for the digestion of starches. But, as you know by now, the whole B complex in some form should be added to prevent imbalances if only one B factor is given.

For simple indigestion, the preceding measures should be of help. To sum up:

—The use of acid: HCL and/or apple cider vinegar

—Soured milks or acidophilus culture to establish or maintain a healthy intestinal flora

—Do not gulp, but Fletcherize your food.

However, this may be only half the story. If your indigestion is due to gall bladder dysfunction, of which you may not be aware, there is still more help for you. We will discuss gall bladder problems next, including some startling surprises as well as how to get rid of gallstones naturally.

REFERENCES
(See *Bibliography* for fuller details.)

1. Horace Fletcher, M.A., *Fletcherism, What It Is*.
2. Linda Clark, *Be Slim and Healthy*.
3. Joseph M. Kadans, N.D., Ph.D., *Modern Encyclopedia of Herbs*.
4. *Potter's New Cyclopaedia*.

18: GALL BLADDER PROBLEMS

An underfunctioning gall bladder can lead to a host of surprising problems. Indigestion, gas, a feeling of fullness, nausea, constipation, a disturbance in your vision (including spots before your eyes, even a cataract), nightmares, and edema of the ankles may result. Other gall bladder symptoms include not only intolerance of fats, but anemia, dizziness or vertigo, bloating, acne, one form of psoriasis and other skin lesions due to inadequate fat absorpotion. Poor gall bladder function can even produce hypoglycemia symptoms such as a craving for sweets, which disappears temporarily when the sweets are eaten.

Conditions associated with gall bladder dysfunction include halitosis, clay-colored or hard dry stools (indicating a lack of bile) and surprisingly, some symptoms usually attributed to a deficiency of the bioflavonoids (Vitamin C complex) such as breakdown of capillaries, varicose veins, phlebitis and hemorrhoids. Even allergies and sneezing attacks have been noted as resulting from a disturbed gall bladder.

Obviously, biliousness and bilious headaches are more or less common, but lesser, symptoms, whereas jaundice is the most extreme result, caused by various conditions, ranging from a virus to a complete stoppage of the bile duct, probably by a gallstone. In chronic gall bladder dysfunction, the skin may be merely a pasty color or may become yellowish; the whites of the eyes, ditto, and the disposition decidedly cranky and irritable. "Watch for the whites of their eyes" could be the watchword for a dysfunctioning gall bladder. If someone snarls at you or bites off your head if you bump into them, suspect their gall bladder! If that same person has, knowingly, or unknowingly corrected his gall bladder problem, which is often possible with a little knowledge, the next time you see him (or her) you will find a sunny, cheerful disposition. Astounding, but true. If that person is you, you will be looking at the world not through murky, but rose colored glasses and feel a *joie de vivre* instead of a "get-out-of-my-way" outlook on life.

Many people get tired putting up with this gall bladder inconvenience and, urged by their doctor, decide to have it removed surgically. Strangely, after a few months of not-so-easy recovery which is often falsely promised by the surgeon, you, *and* the doctor, suddenly realize that the operation did not cure your symptoms; they have all returned. Patients have told me this and even doctors have admitted it, but no one knows why. So a better approach is to learn what causes gall bladder trouble and, as many have already done, do everything you can to solve the problems before submitting to the knife.

Your gall bladder is a small organ, adjacent to your liver, which stores bile and releases it for digestion. A small duct, shaped like a Y, carries the bile, both from the gall bladder and the liver to the intestines, where it is needed to aid digestion. If the flow is insufficient, or the bile has become thick and sluggish or congested, gas, constipation and any of the problems mentioned above may result. Burping, a doctor once told me, *always* means that your gall bladder is acting up.

Bile is supposed to help you digest fat, which includes the fat soluble Vitamins A,D,E, and K. For those people who erroneously decide that the giving up of fat is the answer, I have news for you. You will get worse, not better. Some fat, of the right kind, is absolutely necessary. Why? Without fat you can develop gallstones. And without fat, the fat soluble Vitamins A,E,D, and K, which *must* have fat for their assimilation, cannot be used by your body. If your vision has gone on the blink so that you cannot drive at night, or do sewing or other close-up work, your Vitamin A is probably not being absorbed. If your heart is acting up, your Vitamin E may not be sufficiently provided or absorbed. If your bones ache, your Vitamin D may be unused. And if your whole digestive system is in an uproar, your Vitamin K, which, among other things, regulates your intestinal flora, may be in short supply. So you dare not take a chance by giving up fat and depriving your body of these valuable vitamins.[1]

Many gall bladder sufferers are breakfast skippers, which compounds the problem. You need something solid in the morning, besides juice, coffee and a cigarette, to start your gall bladder churning. The best thing you can take for breakfast is bran in some form. Drs. Neil Painter and Kenneth Heaton of England, state that when a high fibre diet, such as bran is eaten, "it sweeps the degenerated bile salts out of the colon and the vast majority of patients report relief of symptoms."[2]

At breakfast, as well as other meals, you'd better up your protein, and lower your carbohydrate intake, too, since both can cause your body to produce insufficient bile. And one thing leads to another. As you add protein, you may need HCL, or at least some apple cider vinegar in water, with your meals. The late Dr. Royal Lee, a nutrition expert, said, "Hydrochloric acid is very important in all gall bladder cases."

What else can you do to help your gall bladder work better and prevent trouble? The main goal is to keep that bile flowing. Dr. Lee said, "Failure of the mechanism of bile flow may be due to many causes. Many patients considered operable have been restored to a symptom-free basis. Therefore, all essential factors should be tried first."

John E. Eichenlaub, M.D.[3] says, "You can usually get a lazy gall bladder into action simply by taking one or two tablespoons of olive oil before each meal. This starts the flow of bile before the rest of the food enters the stomach. Although you may get a bit more indigestion from the oil for the first few days, you should see marked improvement inside two weeks. . . . A low fat diet (*not* a no-fat diet) helps ward off further attacks of bilious indigestion. Fried foods, pork, rich pastries and gravies, etc., must go. Replace cream with half-and-half, avoid whipping cream and keep butter down to a few pats a day. Eat plenty of lean broiled or boiled meat, vegetables and fruit."[3]

It may be that you cannot begin with as much oil as Dr. Eichenlaub recommends. If not, try less and work upward. Follow the oil with, or take it in, some tart juice and it will be easier to get down. Although all oils help, there seems to be an affinity between olive oil and the gall bladder.

Don't be afraid of eating eggs daily. The yolks contain lecithin. Adelle Davis, during her lifetime, said a great many wise things which were, at the time, laughed at by the medics and scientists. Afterward, they were forced to eat their words. She wrote, "Foods such as yeast, nuts, and unrefined grains, containing B vitamins and/or oils, increase the production of lecithin; and they, as well as lard, stimulate the emptying of the gall bladder, because lecithin breaks cholesterol into tiny particles and keeps it in suspension, a high lecithin content of bile would appear to be vitally important in preventing gallstones."[1]

Sure enough, the greatly respected English medical journal, *Lancet* (May 26, 1956) finally admitted, "Two preventive measures for gallstones are sunflower seeds and brewer's yeast."

Then, *Science News* (April 12, 1969) announced, "Recent studies by two physicians at Ohio State University College of Medicine, show that lecithin, a component of bile that helps dissolve cholesterol, is lower than normal in patients who have had gallstones . . . feeding patients soybean lecithin increases lecithin in the bile and dissolves more cholesterol. The ultimate aim is to learn if soybean lecithin will dissolve existing stones and prevent new ones from forming."

In addition to taking oil and lecithin to speed the flow of bile, there are other natural measures. Beet tops or products derived from them, have been found to increase the bile flow as well as to aid carbohydrate and fat metabolism. Chamomile (also spelled *camomile*) tea made from the plant's blossoms, is reported in one herbal manual as definitely a help in speeding up the flow of bile. Russian black radish tablets (at health stores) appear to do the same thing. One friend was suffering from gall bladder problems and was told by her doctor to, "Watch it: surgery may be necessary!" Since she had just recovered from a long convalescence from surgery as a result of an accident, she said she could not face further surgery. So she tried the natural way.

She drank chamomile tea daily, took Russian black radish tablets, cut down her fat intake of cream, butter, etc., as recommended in Dr. Eichenlaub's statement above. I questioned her three years later and she said that her gall bladder disturbance subsided promptly on this program, and today she has forgotten that she even has a gall bladder.

What Causes Gallstones?

There are different types of gallstones. The cholesterol type is considered the easier type to dissolve. Many people have gallstones and have had them for years. Not until they begin to move out, if they are large, do some people become aware of them. But more about this, shortly. Meanwhile, what causes them in the first place?

Sluggish bile flow can lead to gallstone formation but there are other causes, too. For instance, according to *Lancet* stones could be induced by near starvation diets adopted by those who are trying to lose weight. *Lancet* has also observed that use of The Pill increased not only the risk of blood clots, but gallstones.[4] A deficiency of Vitamin C in guinea pigs also produced gallstones.[5]

Adelle Davis reported that animals deprived of Vitamin E developed gallstones, which dissolved when the E was supplied. She states that low or no fat diets have caused gallstones, due to preventing the gall bladder from emptying completely and causing the bile to become thick and stagnant.[1] A study at Bucknell University confirmed the fact that a fat-free diet caused gallstones in humans.[6] People who are afraid to eat cholesterol foods are also on the wrong track. Dr. Hulda Magalhaes of Bucknell University reported that a cholesterol-free diet caused gallstones in experimental animals.[7]

Gallstones can not only be formed from different substances, but the size can vary tremendously from gravel to the size of a small egg. If the stone is not large, it can pass unnoticed and be expelled during a bowel movement without any discomfort. But sometimes a moderately large gallstone can become lodged in the entrance to the common bile duct where it can cause not only blockage of bile but extreme pain. The pain can come quickly, is known as gallstone colic, and radiates from just under the ribs at the right to the top of the shoulder. It often is accompanied by vomiting and cold sweating and may pass off later when the stone moves through the duct into the bowel, or back into the gall bladder. If the gallstone is trapped, the pain may subside as the muscles in the wall adapt to it. However, the pain may return from time to time, though with less intensity and become a nagging semipermanent problem for which a doctor may prescribe surgery.

Adelle Davis stated that many patients for whom she had planned diets with many nutrients, have passed gallstones with little difficulty. Even if a gallstone gets stuck in the entrance to the common duct, she said, medical intervention has relieved the pain while the stone is passing. The discomfort lasts a few hours, but, she added, "Once forced through the bile duct, it is gone forever." On the other side of the coin, records show that in 1969 alone, 439,000 Americans submitted to gall bladder surgery.

It is possible to live without a gall bladder, but this still means that some fat is necessary for vitamin assimilation. Even the American Medical Association warns against low-fat or fat-free diets because they deprive the individual of, and prevent absorption of, the essential fatty acids, carotene, and Vitamins A, D, E, and K.[1]

Natural Remedies for Gallstones

There is one method not of dissolving, but of *removing* gallstones, providing they are not too large to become lodged in the common duct. I have known both patients and doctors who have used this method, sometimes after ascertaining by X-rays that the stone (or stones) can pass though the duct easily. I heard a chief surgeon of a large New York City hospital suggest this method to a relative of mine, as well as a college friend of his, before trying surgery. The doctor had seen good results when the method had been used by another physician. The method, often called a folk remedy, has· different versions. The most common is as follows:

At bedtime, combine ½ cup of olive oil with ½ cup fresh squeezed lemon or grapefruit juice. Stir vigorously and gulp down the entire mixture without delay. Go to bed immediately and stay there, since nausea may, or may not develop. In the morning, drink a cup of something hot and, if you wish, place a strainer under you when you have the first bowel movement. You may find small pebble-like stones. A variation of this theme substitutes apple juice for the lemon or grapefruit juice, as well as substituting apple juice every two hours for any solid food for two days before taking the oil-juice formula. This approach is said not only to dissolve stones, but to clean out the gall bladder of its old, thick, congested bile as well. The malic acid in the apple juice is given credit for the good effects. However, the oil apparently has value, too.[8,9]

One case history described a man who took one full cup of olive oil at a time and always passed gallstones the next morning. He found that by later taking calcium and magnesium the oil treatment no longer produced gallstones. This may be explained by the magnesium which has also been credited with dissolving kidney stones.[10,7]

Gallstones have been dissolved in rabbits by giving them not olive, but cod liver oil in large quantitites, as reported in a veterinary journal. The dissolving substance in this oil is glyceride.[11]

Less dramatic measures have been used. Adelle Davis has cited studies in which Vitamins A and E have dissolved the old stones, as well as prevented new ones. Don't forget to include lecithin, too, in some form—liquid or granules in your gall bladder for stone removing or prevention program.

And don't sell chamomile tea short! Not only is it reputed to increase the flow of bile, but it has long been known to dissolve gallstones. Culpeper, the herbalist, who lived from 1616 to 1654 wrote, "That it is excellent for the stone, appears in this which I have seen tried, viz., that a stone that hath been taken out of the body of a man, being wrapped in camomile, will in time dissolve, and in a little time, too."[12]

The late Claudia V. James, in her little book, *That Old Green Magic*,[13] tells how a man gave her a few of the sixty-four gallstones he had had removed by surgery. He told her she couldn't dissolve them with chamomile, since he and his wife had been hitting them with a big hammer and couldn't even break them. Claudia James, determined to prove Culpeper's statement, set up her own experiment.

She made a solution of fourteen chamomile flowers (as found in dried tea form at health stores) in one tablespoon of boiling water, poured it into a small glass and dropped two of the gallstones into it. The next day the stones were in four pieces; in five days they were like gravel and in ten days were completely dissolved.

While you are clearing up your gall bladder problem, there are a few other tips: Dr. Eichenlaub says, "Some patients find that they get considerable relief from taking bile salts. One tablet with each meal usually helps to keep the bowels active and prevents some bloating and gas pain."[3] (Bile salts are available separately or in combination with other digestive enzymes at health stores.)

Subsequent research has shown that bile salts should be taken only temporarily, or occasionally, since continued use—at least if made from ox bile—may cause irritation of the gall bladder.

Some doctors believe that gall bladder patients should avoid eating large meals, and Dr. Eichenlaub firmly believes that one should drink enough water. He says, "Drink enough water to ward off thirst. Studies show that gall bladder sufferers seldom put water on the table and drink much less fluid than other people."

One of the main causes of gall bladder disturbance is tension. An example has been reported: a man, a high-powered city executive, contracted gall bladder symptoms only when under stress from his demanding job. Whenever he moved to the country, the gall bladder became normal and remained so until he returned to his city job. The reason: tension can constrict the gall bladder muscles, and this interferes with bile flow.

Dr. Eichenlaub also points out that exercise is a must. He says, "Walk at least two miles a day, or take equivalent amount of other, similar exercise. Lazy gall bladder type indigestion, often followed by stone formation, occurs mainly in people who remain physically inactive."

So there you have it. Pamper your gall bladder and it will pay you handsome rewards.

REFERENCES

(See *Bibliography* for fuller details.)

1. Adelle Davis, *Let's Get Well.*
2. *Here's Health*, Feb., 1973, p. 17.
3. John E. Eichenlaub, M.D., *A Minnesota Doctor's Home Remedies for Common and Uncommon Ailments.*

4. *The New York Times*, July 4, 1973.

5. *Nutrition Abstracts and Reviews*, July, 1969, # 4773.

6. Linda Clark, *Stay Young Longer.*

7. Linda Clark, *Get Well Naturally.*

8. *Here's Health*, December, 1973.

9. Hanna Kroeger, *Old Time Remedies for Modern Ailments*. Also: Paavo Airola, *How To Get Well*.

10. *Prevention*, August, 1969, p. 35.

11. *American Journal of Veterinary Research*, 32: 427–432, 1971.

12. *Culpeper's Complete Herbal*.

13. Claudia V. James, *That Old Green Magic*.

19: HELP FOR HEART TROUBLE

Heart disease has long been considered the No. 1 killer in this country. Yet, surprisingly, according to Dr. Jeremiah Stamler, of Chicago, heart disease has recently been reported as decreasing. Perhaps the reason is that more people are eating wheat germ. Don't laugh; there is laboratory proof that this simple, natural food substance can be a remedy for heart disease. As proof, the Minnesota Agricultural Experiment Station discovered a few years ago that cattle which looked normal and healthy, suddenly began dropping dead of heart disease. Detective work by researchers found the cause; wheat germ, which contains Vitamin E, had been removed from their feed rations. When the wheat germ was restored, the cattle deaths ceased.[1]

Does this apply to cattle only? Definitely not. Two doctors, Wilfrid E. Shute, M.D. and Evan Shute, M.D., both brothers from Canada, have rehabilitated over 30,000 cases of heart disease with Vitamin E. They have returned wheelchair cases to normal living. Even many patients hospitalized after a serious heart attack have gone back to mowing lawns by a push-, not a power-mower. Sufferers from various types of heart disease, including coronary thrombosis, have been improved by Vitamin E therapy.

Wheat germ has been permanently removed from most of the human diet as it was removed only temporarily from the diet of cattle. Why? When the steel roller mill was invented, it replaced the stone grinding process because it was faster, although it impoverished the flour. The heat generated by the mill reduced the protein content and caused the delicate wheat germ to gum up the machinery. So the millers decided to eliminate the wheat germ. To their delight, they also learned that the flour, minus the wheat germ, kept far longer on the grocery shelves without spoiling.

This practice became widespread about 1900. Dr. Wilfrid Shute says, "Prior to the removal of the wheat germ, with its Vitamin E, there were no cases of coronary thrombosis. Now it is one of the nation's major killers. . . . In clinical practice of more than twenty years, involving many thousands of patients, I have found Vitamin E a superb antithrombin (clot dissolver) in the bloodstream. When flour milling underwent the great change around the turn of the century, the Vitamin E in the diet was greatly reduced and with the loss of this natural antithrombin, coronary thrombosis appeared on the scene."[2]

Dr. Shute admits that although coronary thrombosis is not the only form of heart disease, it has caused up to one million deaths per year in the U.S. And he states that Vitamin E is useful in other types of heart disease, both for prevention and treatment. Why does Vitamin E work so well for hearts? There are various reasons, but in addition to the antithrombin factor, the vitamin appears to decrease the need for oxygen in the heart so it can function better and more easily. Vitamin E is also known to improve circulation, and muscle strength. (The heart is a muscle.)

How Much?

How much Vitamin E should be used? The amount is an individual matter. The researchers have learned that the need varies in different people, ranging from 50 to 260 percent.[3] This means that different individuals require different amounts, not only for coronary heart conditions, but for arteriosclerosis, angina, chronic leg ulcers, chronic phlebitis, and many related conditions, all of which have been helped by Vitamin E.[2]

When Vitamin E treatment was announced to the medical profession in the early days of its use, many doctors jumped on the bandwagon and began to use it. Soon, however, they gave up in disgust, insisting that it did not work. The reason was because they used a very tiny dose, usually 30 international units, apparently, on everybody! No wonder they scoffed at the time, and are still scoffing. Yet, this amount is the average RDA (Recommended Dietary Allowance) used today among many orthodox doctors.

Dr. Evan Shute says, "Half a dose of Vitamin E does not do half a job, as we pointed out years ago. One either uses the proper dose for that patient and his particular condition, or one is not using anything. Too small a dose is equivalent to half-treating a diabetic . . . if one is in doubt, it is safer (with two exceptions, noted later) to overtreat than undertreat. *Let us emphasize this point: if you use Vitamin E, use enough.*"[4] (Emphasis mine.)

The Doctors Shute prescribe from 300 I.U. to 2,400 I.U. daily, depending on the circumstances. Without a nutritionally trained doctor to guide you, you may have to feel your way toward establishing your own dosage, as the Shutes do. They often start with 100 or 200 I.U. daily and increase the amount gradually until optimum effects are noted, perhaps cessation of shortness of breath or pain, etc., but before any possible side effects are felt. Dr. Evan Shute believes that there are few people who cannot take 50, or 100, or even 300 I.U. daily. He adds, "We think that the average normal male should take about 600 a day, and the average female 400 I.U. a day."[5]

Vitamin E Antagonists
There are certain antagonists to Vitamin E, and you should

not take them simultaneously with Vitamin E. The antagonists are female hormones (estrogen), inorganic iron, and chlorine. If you take the hormones or inorganic iron, the solution to the problem is easy. Merely take Vitamin E at breakfast time, and the other substances at evening dinner. Separating the antagonists from the vitamin intake by eight to twelve hours will apparently protect you. Chlorine can be removed from your drinking water by boiling it, or leaving it overnight at room temperature to evaporate before refrigerating it. And one more tip: Dr. Shute says that if you should temporarily stop taking Vitamin E, it will disappear entirely from your bloodstream after three days.[2]

Even if you have satisfied these requirements, you still may be taking Vitamin E and not absorbing it. Vitamin E is a fat soluble vitamin and if you are on a fat-free diet, or even a very low fat diet, your body cannot dissolve the vitamin so that you can use it properly. Even if you add extra fat such as the polyunsaturates, you may run into trouble. This is because the polyunsaturates in the diet increase the rate of oxidation of Vitamin E. In case you have decided by this time you can't win, all you have to do is, if you increase your amount of polyunsaturates, also increase your amount of Vitamin E.[3]

Is Too Much Vitamin E Dangerous?

According to Dr. Wilfrid Shute, there is danger in taking too much Vitamin E in two conditions only: high blood pressure, or if you have a history of rheumatic fever. In both cases, he recommends the same procedure: the amount of Vitamin E should be started cautiously at a low level and increased very gradually. He suggests that you start with 90 I.U. daily for one month, 120 I.U. daily for the second month; and 150 I.U. daily for the third month. If high blood pressure is already established and you take too much at first, it may send the pressure higher. You will eventually find the right dose for you at which point your heart symptoms subside, or your blood pressure remains steady. One nutritionist I know has found that she cannot go higher than 400 I.U. daily because it always raises her blood pressure. So she remains content on that dosage, which is the average recommended for females as it happens. Yet, for others, Vitamin E has reduced high blood pressure.

As for those who have been rheumatic fever patients, Dr. Shute believes that they should rarely go higher than 300 I.U. daily, since more may lead to fatal results.[2]

For those doctors who object to a patient's self-treatment, Dr. Shute answers, "Of course people shouldn't treat themselves, [but] . . . fortunately, the average patient has more to gain by treating himself than he has to lose by poor selection of a doctor. This is one reason why we have always been anxious to get this knowledge into medical hands. But if medical hands continue to reject it, what alternative is there left but for patients to treat themselves, as they are already doing by the hundreds of thousands?"[6]

What Type of Vitamin E is Best?

Different types of Vitamin E listed on labels are explained in my book, *Know Your Nutrition*.[5] (Due to lack of space, I cannot repeat the entire explanation here.) The book tells which types are natural, which are synthetic. Some people believe the natural variety is best. However, the Shutes used a certain brand of synthetic E before turning to a natural brand, and achieved success. (The name of this brand has not been publicized, possibly because it is no longer available.) The Shutes also used a form of Vitamin E called alpha tocopherol. This is one factor, only, of the whole family or E complex discovered later. The complex in-includes the alpha, beta, gamma, and delta tocopherols, and many researchers believe the mixed tocopherols, as they are called, are more effective.

In some cases, Vitamin E is manufactured in a water (not fat) dispersible form, designed for those who have trouble digesting fats. But many nutritionists believe that some fat is needed by the body for proper functioning of the gall bladder.

It is also true that some people are allergic to wheat and wheat germ as well as to wheat germ oil, from which much Vitamin E is extracted. In this case, the dry powdered form of E, available in capsules, is suggested for those allergic to wheat products.

In any case, Vitamin E, which is now considered a heart-saving, and thus a life-saving, vitamin, is the most expensive of all vitamins. The amount found in multiple vitamin supplements is considered by nutritionists too low for the average person. Since adding more would raise the cost for the manufacturer, thus the price to the consumer, it is better to get your own Vitamin E separately.

And if you value your life, you will realize that the price is well worth it. There are many interesting case histories cited in *Ailing and Healthy Hearts*, written by Wilfrid E. Shute, M.D., with Harald J. Taub. Anyone with a heart problem should read every word of this enlightening book.[2]

A heart patient sent me an account of his own case. He was found by a doctor to have a heart "off beat"; the doctor sent him from specialist to specialist and eventually to a hospital where he spent three months in bed, all to no avail. After reading a book about Vitamin E for hearts, this patient purchased a bottle of Vitamin E. After taking only 600 I.U., he wrote me that as early as the following day, his "off-beat" heart became regular, emitting the normal lubb-dup, lubb-dup sound. He tells me that it has been regular ever since, although he was past eighty-five at the time of writing me; he had also worked all the time, and was well in every way with a blood pressure reading of 134/74.

Other Causes and Treatments of Heart Disease

There is a well-publicized study of heart disease known as the Framingham (Massachusetts) study. This study involved 5,127 volunteers ranging from ages thirty to sixty-two. The study reported (according to their findings) six factors or causes of heart disease. They were:

1. Cholesterol increase (considered the greatest threat)
2. High blood pressure (to be discussed in the next chapter)
3. Heavy smoking

4. Lowered vitality
5. Heart malfunction is noted by an electrocardiogram
6. Overweight

You will notice that there is not one word in the findings of this study mentioning *diet* or nutritional *deficiency* as a cause! Yet Vitamin E deficiency has already been noted and there are other dietary deficiencies which have also been found to affect hearts. If these deficiencies are overcome, studies show that the heart function has improved. Here are some deficiency examples:

Deficiency of Vitamin C complex reduces the capacity of the blood stream to carry oxygen to the heart.[7] Vitamin C complex also protects against capillary fragility which can lead to strokes.[7A]

B vitamins affect the nerves, to which the heart is extremely sensitive. Vitamin B-1 has been specifically cited in this respect, but all B vitamins must accompany the use of one factor.[8]

Vitamin B-6 not only helps the body use fat more efficiently, but regulates the sodium-potassium balance, which controls edema.[9]

Folic Acid (another B vitamin)[10]

A deficiency of protein. The heart is a muscle made of protein, which must be replaced constantly in the diet for heart repair and maintenance.[11]

A deficiency of trace minerals such as iodine, copper, manganese, and zinc, as well as calcium for calming purposes.[12]

There is further testimony of the effect of nutrients on hearts. According to Dr. E. G. Knox as reported in *Lancet* (June 30, 1973), a lack of Vitamin C is a factor in heart attacks as well as strokes. Dr. Knox stated that the more Vitamin C there is in the diet, the less likely a fatal heart attack or stroke is apt to occur.

Dr. Emil Ginter, of the Institute of Bratislava, Czechoslovakia, has found that Vitamin C also protects against high blood cholesterol.

The New York Times (March 7, 1973) reported, "Judicious supplements of trace minerals, vitamins and hormones, used by a group of physicians in Baltimore, Maryland, and Atlanta, Georgia, reduced mortality and recurrence of heart attacks in 25 patients whom they had treated for six years. There were no new cases of angina. None of the patients had to be admitted to hospitals for complications or coronary thrombosis, which means obstruction of the important heart artery."

Too much of something can be as devasting as too little. As an example, carbohydrates, especially sugar, are contraindicated for hearts. John Yudkin, M.D., Department of Nutrition, Queen Elizabeth College, London University, England,[13] believes that sugar is a major cause of heart disease. He cites the rise of coronary deaths in England which paralleled the rise in sugar consumption, whereas tribes in other parts of the world, though on a high fat diet, but low in sugar, have virtually no heart disease. Dr. Yudkin believes that sugar which, except for calories, contains *no nutrients,* should be banned and that there should be a law against giving children candy.

The Truth About Cholesterol

We have been so deluged with warnings about cholesterol that it has become a household word and everyone seems scared out of his wits at the very mention of it. The problem is that there is a great misunderstanding among doctors and patients alike. Cholesterol is not a no-no, but a goodie! If you don't believe it, read on. But first we have to understand the meaning of two words we also hear so much about: arteriosclerosis and atherosclerosis. The first, *arterio*sclerosis, is often called "hardening of the arteries." Actually this is a thickening and narrowing of the arteries due to a decrease of elasticity of the artery walls. On the other hand, *athero*sclerosis is a filling up and clogging of the arteries with substances such as fat and cholesterol, which prevents the blood from efficiently reaching various parts of the body.

It is at this point that the misunderstanding begins. Cholesterol is registered in the blood and gives an index to what is going on in the rest of the body. The number given you when your cholesterol is determined means the amount of cholesterol measured in milligrams, per 100 cc of blood. In other words, a cholesterol reading of 240 means you have 240 milligrams of cholesterol in approximately 100 cc of blood. In Americans, if the reading is higher than 240 (150–180 is safer) this indicates that arteries affecting eyes, legs, feet and hands as well as the heart are all not receiving their optimum quota of blood, due to clogging. This may indeed indicate trouble ahead. But the misunderstanding comes not from the fact that the condition exists, but what is to be done about it.

The average doctor immediately tells a patient with a high cholesterol level to eliminate fats and all cholesterol foods, usually eggs, liver, butter, and other foods which are, it is true, high in cholesterol but also highly nutritious!

Yet, Ruth Winter points out, "Many clinicians believe—and the Framingham study seems to bear it out—that people so inclined physiologically will manufacture cholesterol in their blood no matter what they eat."[6] Others agree. Drs. E. Cheraskin and W.M. Ringsdorf, Jr., state that eighty percent of the cholesterol in the blood is manufactured by the body, and the remaining twenty percent in the diet is not significant in the development of atherosclerosis for the majority. In fact, other researchers have gone so far as to say that since the body needs cholesterol to nourish various glands and assist other body functions, the less cholesterol given, the more furiously the body manufactures it to make up the deficit.[14]

Then there is the fat furor. Saturated fat is considered a dirty word, whereas unsaturated fat is extolled from the housetops. But this concept has also been distorted and converted into a scare story which many experts refuse to believe.

You will notice that Dr. Yudkin has pointed out that many tribes with a low incidence of heart disease, have had a *high* consumption of animal fat (saturated) and butter, though low in sugar. Dr. George Christakis, a director of the New York Bureau of Nutrition, has stated that fatal heart attacks in men on a low fat diet are actually only forty percent among those eating an average American diet, usually high in fat and cholesterol. I remember Carlton Fredericks, who may be the most learned living nutritionist of our time, saying over twenty years ago that the day would come when the theory of natural saturated (animal) fat vs. unsaturated fat as being dangerous would be disproved. Others are beginning to agree.

The sensible approach is not to worry about the fat problem, but to learn what to do about it.

Fortunately, as Adelle Davis and others have shown us, atherosclerosis, or high cholesterol in the blood, *can* be reversed. The plugged arteries can be unplugged by a simple change in the diet. Lecithin, a food substance made from the soy bean, is an emulsifier for both fat and cholesterol and can dissolve both in the body. Angina, one type of heart disease, which may be caused by atherosclerosis, has yielded to lecithin and I know personally one case where this happened.[15]

Adelle Davis has stated, "Even when atherosclerosis is far advanced, health is restored after lecithin is supplied in the diet. . . . Many physicians have successfully reduced blood cholesterol with lecithin. For example, 4 to 6 tablespoons (of soy lecithin in granules, available at health stores) have been given daily to patients who had suffered heart attacks and had been consistently resistant to many cholesterol-lowering medications, some as long as ten years." Adelle added that although no other dietary changes were made, the level of blood cholesterol dropped within three months, the patients were more energetic, were relieved of pain and other symptoms, and had a greater capacity for work.[16]

Although Adelle used the soy lecithin granules, others use liquid lecithin with excellent results, believing that a teaspoon taken morning and night keeps lecithin in solution in the bloodstream at all times.[17]

If you take lecithin, be sure to step up your calcium intake. Lecithin is high in phosphorus, which combines with calcium and is excreted from the body. If you do not already have sufficient calcium, the result may be a calcium deficiency leading to leg cramps, or cramps in other parts of your body including the intercostal muscles (rib cage) which is sometimes mistaken for a heart attack, but is not. Calcium also soothes the heart, so be sure you have enough.

Adelle told me a story of a small girl from an affluent pineapple family in Hawaii, who was bedridden with a cholesterol level of 600. Doctors did not expect her to recover or return to school. Adelle promptly recommended six tablespoons of lecithin granules daily, in juice, on salads, etc., and within three months the child's cholesterol was not only normal, she was back at school!

There are other ways to outwit high cholesterol. A spoonful of garlic was reported as beneficial by *Lancet,* the English medical journal, who reported that two garlic capsules (equivalent to 50 mg. of fresh garlic) could be a great protection against excess fat in the blood which otherwise might lead to blood clots and arterial disease. Volunteers with high cholesterol were found to show a drop in cholesterol within three hours after taking garlic and their blood was "thinner" than usual.[18]

George Thosteson, M.D., the American medical newspaper columnist, does not worry about a special diet for high cholesterol sufferers. He merely asks his patients to lose weight, which, he says, takes care of the problem.

Another cholesterol-lowering solution was reported from Louisiana State University, which stated that no matter what you eat, whether your diet is high in fats or your cholesterol is high, regular exercise will reduce it to normal. This study was confirmed by Dr. Alfredo Lopez, professor of medicine at the same university, who found that in examining 100 men, the greater the physical fitness, the lower the cholesterol.[19]

Some Surprising Causes of Heart Trouble

The heart is a hard-working organ, yet is very sensitive to many things you might not expect. Here are some examples:

1. *Homogenized milk.* Dr. Kurt A. Oster, chief cardiologist at Park City Hospital, Bridgeport, Conn., believes that the milk

homogenization process breaks down the fat and an enzyme, Xantine Oxidase, into tiny particles which, instead of being digested, enter the blood stream. The large fat globules in regular cow's milk (untreated) are not a problem, he says, because they are apparently digested. Even 99% fat-free milk is a hazard, if homogenized, Dr. Oster claims. Finland, with the highest death rate from heart disease as well as being noted for the highest milk consumption, is a possible example. The United States, though with a relatively low milk consumption, uses mostly homogenized milk.[20]

2. *Coffee.* "It's terrible but delicious stuff," says Dr. William J. Lukash, National Medical Center, Bethesda, Md. Among *heavy coffee drinkers*, Dr. Lukash states, it causes headaches, nervousness, indigestion, diarrhea, and worst of all, heart attacks.[21]

3. *Water.* Some types of water contribute to heart disease, according to many international studies. In London, England, a study cited in *Lancet* reported: "Men living in areas where the drinking water is hard, live longer and are less likely to have strokes and coronary-artery disease. There is evidence that some component of hard water, possibly calcium, is responsible."[22]

Erwin Di Cyan, Ph.D., a scientist and nutrition reporter says, "Water is soft when it is relatively free from calcium and magnesium. Soft water is reported by some to cause hardening of the arteries, or arteriosclerosis (not atherosclerosis)."[23]

For those who have water softeners, the solution is to attach the softener to the hot water only, and drink, either heated or cold, the *un*softened water taken from the untreated cold water tap.

Scientists of the World Health Organization (W.H.O.) convening at Geneva, Switzerland, also confirmed that there is a definite trend toward greater occurrence of heart attacks in populations using soft water, than in those areas relying on hard water. These range from soft-water cities such as Glasgow, Scotland and Winston-Salem, North Carolina, to hard-water cities such as London and Omaha. Not only do W.H.O. scientists believe that there are protective minerals in the hard water, but that the soft, acid water can leach out lead, and cadmium from tap water pipes. Distilled water, they report, is 100% soft. Hard water is not corrosive, so carries less hazard in this connection.[24]

Meanwhile, Henry A. Schroeder, M.D., world famous trace mineral researcher, warns against the serious toxicity of lead and cadmium in water delivered into the house through water pipes.[25] The suggestion has been made that one should allow the water to run for some seconds in the morning, before using it for beverages or cooking. Water standing in the pipes during the night can increase the concentration of these heavy, toxic metals.

There is one further possible hazard from water: chlorine. Joseph M. Price, M.D. learned from experiments with chickens, that those given highly chlorinated water became lethargic, exhibited frayed and dirty feathers, and pale, dropping combs. These chickens died spontaneously and on autopsy 95% were found to have damaged aortas and atherosclerosis. The control group which were not given highly chlorinated water did not die and maintained rigorous health.[26]

As stated earlier, the easiest way to remove chlorine is to boil water or let it stand at room temperature overnight to evaporate the chlorine before refrigerating and using the water.

There are some nutritional supplements for protection against the heavy metals suggested in my book, *Know Your Nutrition.*[5]

4. *Tobacco.* Apparently there is no argument that tobacco is one of the major causes of heart attacks. The three most damaging elements of cigarette smoke believed to be hazardous to hearts and contributing to an attack, are carbon monoxide, nicotine, and tobacco "tar." Robert Illa, M.D., of Stanford University Medical Staff, calls attention to the U.S. Surgeon General's warning that smoking may be a major risk in heart disease. "Cigarette smokers have a higher death rate from cerebrovascular disease than nonsmokers. Cigarette smoking is associated with a significant increase in atherosclerosis of the aorta and coronary arteries."

Dr. Illa states that carbon monoxide can come from automobile exhaust or air pollution, as well as collect in enclosed places filled with cigarette smoke. He says it is dangerous because it reduces the amount of oxygen reaching the tissues.[27]

Researchers from the Medical College of Wisconsin add, "Tobacco is the single most important factor leading to high carbon monoxide levels."[28] Wilhelm Raab, M.D., believes that nicotine also causes a lack of oxygen in the heart muscles, which can lead to death of the affected tissue.[29]

But the most unexpected effect of smoking has been found in nonsmokers! True, the smoker, himself, is apparently slowly poisoning himself, but those toward whom he blows his smoke are also likely candidates for heart and other major disturbances. Children have even been endangered by smoking parents. Don Matchan has described these hazards and how to avoid them.[27] Many suggestions are offered (and are already being followed by some angry groups of nonsmokers). The suggestions include banning smoking in public places and reinforcing bans on planes, trains and buses except in areas reserved for smokers. This nonsmoker hazard is daily becoming a greater and greater threat. So if someone is blowing smoke in your face, speak up and defend yourself from his thoughtlessness.

Many a case of indigestion is mistaken for a heart attack. Digestive enzymes, especially HCL, taken after each meal, can easily prevent this problem. Digestive enzymes are available at health stores.

The Effect of Stress on the Heart

Stress is probably our biggest heart problem. It can constrict muscles, including the heart muscle, interfere with circulation needed by the heart, and can even raise the cholesterol level. Internal Revenue workers have been found to have a higher cholesterol during the months of income tax preparation, prior to April 15, than at any other time of the year.[15]

Studies galore reveal that stress is related to heart disease, attacks and death, whereas other studies show that tribes which are tranquil, though physically active, have no evidence of heart disease.[30]

Recent studies conducted by religious, industrial and university groups reveal that people who go to church are happier and have fewer heart attacks.[31]

A "bombshell" finding by Drs. Ray H. Rosenman and Meyer Friedman, at Mount Zion Hospital and Medical Center, San Francisco, resulted from a continuing two-and-a-half year study in which 3,000 men, who were classified by personality or behavior, upset all predictions. The men were classified as Type A: overly ambitious and aggressive, and as Type B: calmer, quieter and more unobtrusive. The scientists found a four-fold higher risk of heart disease in the Type A group.[31]

How do you outwit stress? I know a business executive, Type A, who worked day and night, traveled from coast to coast, and became lax about his nutrition, although he knew better. He ended up with not one heart attack, but two, and was hospitalized. On his release, he turned over a new leaf, decided to work less, relax more, do things he liked as well as things he felt obliged to do. He also improved his nutrition. He not only survived, he felt better and looked younger. He became a Type B rather than a Type A. He decided, whenever possible, instead of pushing himself beyond his endurance, to adopt the south-of-the-border *mañana* attitude. He also took more exercise, the kind he enjoyed, such a golfing, tennis, and walking.

R. W. Holderby, M.D., says, "We should have twenty minutes of perspiring exercise daily to burn the sludge out of our blood vessels. Park your car at a distance. Walk to work, walk at lunch time, before breakfast, anytime, but *make* yourself walk."

Dr. Holderby summarizes his own suggestions for preventing a heart attack:

Eat Natural food, grown on fertile soil, fresh and poison-free.
Take vitamin E capsules daily.
Take lecithin granules daily.
Eat enough protein.

Avoid sugar, white flour and other carbohydrates.

Take more exercise.

Don't use tobacco.

Cut down on stress.

A siesta is another way to outwit stress, but unfortunately it is losing favor and becoming outmoded in some countries. The reason: no one has figured out how it can be made to show a financial profit. However, without a siesta, the body is forced to work harder and may not work as efficiently or last as long.

Martha Weinman Lear, reporter to *The New York Times*, said, "The siesta, bless its lazy heart, has no vitamins at all. It just has heart, doing nothing for the blood but making people feel good. Like the overstuffed chair, the bubble bath and other lost and lovely causes, it is personal rather than productive, comfortable rather than functional. It is also remarkably conducive to the warm and steady flow of all the human juices.

"While other countries are outmoding the siesta, we feel America should adopt it. The executive or office worker should be allowed to put his feet on the desk and take forty winks after lunch, or at coffee-break time. The housewife should make it a *rule*. As one industrial physician has remarked, 'For health purposes, the siesta is a swell idea'."

Even if you have had a heart attack, it is not too late to revise your life style and your diet, according to suggestions given in this chapter. Scientists at Harvard School of Public Health proved by laboratory tests with dogs, that following a heart attack, a damaged heart can completely recover and be as good as new. This applies to people too. Cardiologist Dr. Michael Gordon of the University of Miami Medical School also states that the human heart can recover after an attack and the patient can resume a normal life.

REFERENCES
(See *Bibliography* for fuller details.)

1. T. Gullickson and C. Calvery, "Cardiac Failure on Vitamin-free

Reactions as Revealed by Electrocardiograms," Minnesota Experiment Station, *Science*, p. 312, October, 1946.

2. Wilfrid E. Shute, M.D., with Harald J. Taub, *Vitamin E for Ailing and Healthy Hearts*.

3. C. B. Houchin and H. S. Mattil, *Proceedings for Society of Experimental Biology and Medicine*, 50:216, 1942.

4. *Prevention*, p. 86, May, 1971.

5. Linda Clark, *Know Your Nutrition*.

6. Ruth Winter, *Vitamin E, The Miracle Worker*.

7. *Science Newsletter*, August, 1941.

7a. Irwin Stone, *The Healing Factor: Vitamin C Against Disease*.

8. *Chemical Abstracts*, 32, 7:2577, April 10, 1938.

9. John M. Ellis, M.D., with James Presley, *Vitamin B-6, The Doctor's Report*.

10. Journal of the American Geriatric Society, 13: 10, 935–937, October, 1965.

11. E. Cheraskin, M.D., W. M. Ringsdorf, Jr., D.M.D., and J. W. Clark, D.D.S., *Diet and Disease*.

12. James P. Isaacs, M.D., Johns Hopkins School of Medicine; also *American Heart Journal*, 68, 768, 1962.

13. John Yudkin, M.D., Sweet and Dangerous.

14. Edward R. Pinckney, M.D. and Cathey Pinckney, *The Cholesterol Controversy*. See also: Bernard Bellew, M.D. and Joeva Bellew, "The Great Cholesterol Myth Debunked," *Let's Live*, October, 1974; E. Cheraskin, M.D., and W.M. Ringsdorf, D.M.D., with Arline Brecher, *Psychodietetics*.

15. Linda Clark, *Stay Young Longer*.

16. Adelle Davis, *Let's Get Well*.

17. Linda Clark, *Secrets of Health and Beauty*.

18. Reported in *Here's Health*, English health publication, August, 1974.

19. *Rodale's Health Bulletin*, July 10, 1971.

20. *Consumers' Research*, August, 1974.

21. *San Francisco Chronicle*, June 25, 1974.

22. *Ibid*, August 21, 1968.

23. Erwin Di Cyan, Ph.D., *Vitamins in Your Life and the Micronutrients*.

24. *The New York Times*, March 7, 1973.

25. Henry A. Schroeder, M.D., *The Trace Elements and Man.*

26. Joseph M. Price, M.D., *Coronaries, Cholesterol, Chlorine*.

27. Don Matchan, "The Case for the Non-Smoker," *Let's Live*, May, June and July, 1974.

28. *The New York Times*, December 20, 1973.

29. Independent Citizens Research Foundation (ICRF), "Wake Up and Earn a Healthy Heart," Ardsley, N.Y. October 10, 1966.

30. Meyer Friedman, M.D., and Ray H. Rosenman, M.D., *Type A Behavior and Your Heart*.

31. ICRF, "First International Conference on Preventive Cardiology," October, 1964.

20: HIGH BLOOD PRESSURE

(PLEASE NOTE: The information in this chapter is not intended to replace the diagnosis of a medical doctor, but to give you some self-help information in addition to that obtained from the doctor.)

High blood pressure (known to physicians as hypertension) is nothing to play around with. I do not like books or articles that scare the daylights out of you, saying that if you don't do this or that, it is curtains for you. In my opinion, such information may frighten a patient, create more tension, and cause a higher reading than before. High blood pressure is not a disease, but a symptom of existing circulation problems which *may* cause heart attacks, strokes or other disabling conditions, including but not limited to detachment of retina, if not eliminated. Fortunately, when the causes of high blood pressure are removed, both the high blood pressure and the resulting dangers may disappear.[1]

So it behooves you to learn what high blood pressure is, its symptoms, what causes it, and how to handle it, especially in your particular case. While there are general rules which serve as a common denominator, there also are individual variations which may make your case different from others.

There are 30,000,000 cases of high blood pressure in America, and 15,000,000 don't know they have it.[2] Armed with knowledge on how to cope with it, you can relax and stop worrying. There are many things which have helped others to recover and can help you, too. With proper therapy, high blood pressure can almost always be controlled, adding years to your life, and providing better health as well as peace of mind.

What is High Blood Pressure?

There is nothing very mysterious about high blood pressure. The arteries, each somewhat like a garden hose, can narrow through constriction or tension or become plugged with various deposits. Yet the blood still must be pumped through them to the heart and other parts of the body. As the arteries narrow, the blood is squeezed through less space, and the pressure is correspondingly increased.

Or, when larger amounts of water than normal are retained in the body—a condition known as edema—the increased blood volume causes elevated pressure. Yet normal blood pressure is absolutely necessary for normal blood circulation. Why? The heart pumps the blood through the arteries, first into the main artery called the aorta, which branches into smaller arteries, and then into still smaller arteries, finally reaching tiny blood vessels known as capillaries. From there it flows into the veins and back into the heart. The heart pumps 1,440 gallons of blood a day.[1] If there is resistance of any kind in the arteries, the heart becomes overworked in order to keep up the circulation.

Doctors can measure your blood pressure painlessly by using a device which you probably can recognize but cannot pronounce (it is a sphygmomanometer). It is merely a narrow flat rubber bag which is wrapped around your upper arm and inflated with a rubber bulb. A physician listens to your pulse sounds with a stethoscope while he watches the rise of a column of mercury which registers two measurements. These measurements are presented somewhat like a mathematical fraction. The upper number registers your systolic pressure; the lower figure your diastolic pressure. The systolic reading (upper figure) records pressure during the contraction or squeezing period of the heart pump at work; the diastolic (lower figure) pressure is that maintained during the relaxation or resting period of the heart. Depending on age, and other conditions unique to the individual, the normal pressure is considered approximately 135/80. Moderately high blood pressure is 150/100 to 180/100. A reading above that *may* indicate risk. Some women tend to tolerate higher pressures than men.[2]

What Your Arteries Tell

As most people grow older, their arteries supposedly change. In one condition, known as *arteriosclerosis,* or "hardening of the arteries," the walls of the arteries may become thickened and lose their elasticity so that they do not "give" with each heart beat. This places an added burden on the heart pump. In this condition, the inner lining of the arteries may have become rough and corrugated, whereas they were formerly smooth and glistening. Or scar tissue may appear; or hard deposits or blood clots may form on the inner artery walls.

On the other hand, *atherosclerosis* is the condition where the *inside* of the arteries becomes plugged with various deposits, and the blood flow is slowed as the plugging increases.

As either condition progresses, the blood pressure builds up so that in times of extreme exertion or excitement, a bursting point may occur. When a "small stroke" occurs, that is nature's way of telling you to change your life style without any argument! By doing so you can begin to aid nature to eliminate the causes so that the body may control your condition and you can live a joyous life.

Look over the following checklist of symptoms of high blood pressure to see if you recognize any in yourself. If you do, don't panic. Welcome the opportunity to start reversing the condition, rather than worrying about it. Remember, too, as you read the symptoms, that imagination can play havoc if you will let it, like the man who read the medical dictionary and decided he had every disease in the book except "housemaid's knee." Many of these symptoms may be due to some other cause. Even so, it is time to take stock. Natural treatments are available to often help you out of the dilemma.

Some Usual Symptoms of High Blood Pressure

Recurring nosebleeds (actually a safety valve to relieve pressure).

Red blotches of hemorrhages in whites of the eyeballs.

Pounding headache, the most common symptom. It may appear in different areas of head and neck. It may also be a full, tight feeling in or around your head.

Aches and pains of unknown origin elsewhere: arms, shoulder blades, leg, back, etc. Some people assume that this is arthritis.

Dizziness. May be continuous as in vertigo, or be fleeting, such as when you lean over to pick up something.

A feeling of swaying, sometimes as if about to faint (which rarely happens).

Ankle swelling.

Ear noises, or ringing in the ears.

Skin flushing.

Heart palpitations.

Pain in heart regions.

Frequent urination.

Nervous tension and fatigue.

Crossness.

Emotional upsets. In women, a tendency to tears, often associated with menopause.

Tiredness and wakefulness. Insomnia. General restlessness. Waking up "tired."

Falling asleep but waking very early in the morning with pounding or throbbing in head and ears.

Doctors believe that there are two types of blood pressure: primary, or essential; and secondary. Essential hypertension is considered the real thing, whereas secondary hypertension is very often a side effect of some other disturbance in the body.

Causes

Be prepared for some surprises about causes of high blood pressure. Even your doctor may not be familiar with these.

High blood pressure can vary from day to day, week to week, according to temperament, physical activity, rest, certain foods, pain, stress, and other factors.

Weather may influence blood pressure. In some cases, it has been found to be higher in cold weather, lower in warm weather.[3]

Altitude may raise blood pressure. One person had a rise of 60 points within four hours after going to an altitude of 7,000 feet.[4]

Some people with essential hypertension are dynamic, hard driving, nonprocrastinating workers (see Heart Problems for Type A patients). This is the racehorse type of individual whose adrenal glands, usually reserved for sudden emergencies, are mobilized so often that they can't slow down or stop overfunctioning. This type of hypertension patient develops a chronic state of adrenal overfunction, which, like the tired horse, constantly pushes himself beyond his endurance.[3]

Some hypertension is due to imbalance in the acid-alkaline ratio, usually too little acid.

Both food and environment can cause high blood pressure. "People living under natural conditions, eating simple, natural foods, don't have high blood pressure. It is unknown among native races. High blood pressure is often a degenerative condition, due to our 'civilized' diet and our so-called 'civilized' way of life."[1]

For hypertension due to nervous tension and emotional stress, a deficiency of the B vitamins (the entire B complex), calcium and magnesium may be a factor. These nutrients calm nerves and muscles.

Sedentary living (lack of exercise).

The Pill. Women with normal blood pressure have often developed high blood pressure within one to six months after beginning The Pill.[6] A report published by the *Journal of the American Medical Association* involved the collaborative efforts of doctors at ninety-one hospitals in twelve cities, which showed that the birth control pill alone can increase the chance of a stroke.

Soft water, both natural and artificially softened. Residents of soft water areas the world over have been found to have an average of higher blood pressure than those with hard water.[7]

Obesity.

Smoking. A Massachusetts study showed that male cigarette smokers had three times as many strokes (associated with hypertension) as nonsmokers.[5]

Diabetes.

Kidney malfunction.

Cadmium, a toxic metal, is a more recent pollutant which has definitely been found in laboratory experiments to cause high blood pressure. It is found in air, tobacco, soft water, milk and refined grains. According to Henry A. Schroeder, M.D., an expert researcher on the subject, drinking above five cups of coffee or tea daily *doubles* the daily intake of cadmium.[8] One survey found that cadmium was found in forty percent of 720 samples of drinking water from reservoirs and rivers. Cadmium also accumulates as it stands in galvanized or plastic water pipes. In your home, let your water run at least a full minute before using for food preparation or drinking.

In addition to cadmium, nitrates in diet or drinking water can raise blood pressure according to the University of Oregon Medical School.[9] Nitrates together with nitrites (even more dangerous) are found not only in soil and water, but are deliberately added to smoked fish and to *all* ham, bacon, sausage, salami, cold cuts, and hot dogs. These additives are used as preservatives as well as to color the foods to make them look more appetizing. Read your labels!

Coffee and cola drinks, even painkillers which contain caffeine, can raise blood pressure. In large amounts, the caffeine also appears to cause fluid retention. Those with high blood pressure are counseled to avoid these beverages.[10]

Sodium chloride (common table salt) in excess tends to cause edema or fluid retention and raise blood pressure.[11]

Food allergies, especially wheat, for a growing number of people. Other allergies, including milk, have also been found to raise blood pressure in some people.[12]

Hypoglycemia (low blood sugar).

On-again, off-again reducing diets and weight-reducing pills.[13]

Although Dr. Melvin E. Page, an endocrinologist, believes that arteries may be a factor in hypertension, he also believes that the underlying cause is a maladjusted glandular system. He has told me that when the glandular system is in proper balance, and the body chemistry is in perfect adjustment, he finds it almost impossible for the patient to have high blood pressure.[14]

Treatments

Do not be surprised if your doctor does not agree with many of the following treatments, which are natural, not drug oriented. Your doctor was taught only drug treatments in medical school. Although drugs may temporarily alleviate high blood pressure and therefore may in emergencies save lives, they do not *cure* the condition, according to Richard E. Herndon, M.D., Fellow of the American College of Physicians, who wrote in his book on essential hypertension, "No drug treatment is yet known which has ever cured or arrested the progress of essential hypertension, although their temporary palliative value, especially in the early stages, cannot be questioned."[1] The Australian publication in which this statement was quoted, added, "We know of no single instance where the long term effect of drug treatment gave lasting benefit once the drug was discontinued ... yet with the natural treatments (outlined below), high blood pressure can be overcome and IS being overcome. It is up to you."[1]

However, natural treatments do not produce overnight results; they need time to re-educate the body which, given the proper materials, is constantly renewing itself. Medical diagnosis can be valuable, and even a temporary drug, if absolutely necessary, may be a lifesaver while the body is being re-educated.

There are many things not yet clear about high blood pressure, so it is not surprising that medical opinions differ on the interpretation of the systolic (upper figure) and the diastolic (lower figure) readings. The former belief was that the systolic reading was supposed to be 100 plus your present age. This is no longer generally accepted. Many doctors believe that the diastolic reading is the more important, while others believe that the difference between the two is important.

The late Dr. Royal Lee, a nutrition expert, greatly admired for his knowledge by his peers, believed that the important consideration in high blood pressure, was not so much the desired rate of fall in the blood pressure (which varies) but therapy which would take the stress off the organs and tissues involved (described later).

Most doctors lump both readings together and prescribe the same measures for various patients, whether needed or not. For example, too much of the *wrong* kind of salt has been found to cause edema and raise blood pressure. A friend of mine recently visited her doctor who found her blood pressure high and automatically warned her to go on a salt-free diet even though she had no edema at all!

A New Breakthrough?

I found during my research that most books on high blood pressure by physicians repeat each other. The same causes and treatments have been accepted for years and the message is repeated over and over, like a broken record.

However, I came across a surprising new theory from a nutritional therapist who had worked for thirteen years with a specialist on hypertension in countless patients. This thorough study revealed that the *systolic* rise in blood pressure indicated overstimulation of some kind in the body: emotional stress, exciting foods, beverages, even allergies and toxins. A rise in *diastolic* pressure was found to reflect the congestion due to deposits clogging the walls of the arteries. Since what affects one part of the body may automatically affect another, there might be a slight rise in the diastolic, which follows the systolic rise, but for the most part, the study showed that the major rise, due to stimulants, will be registered in the systolic. This provides tremendous help in pinpointing the causes as well as the treatment. So if your systolic is higher than normal, try cutting down on spices, stimulating beverages such as coffee, even alcohol. Also, cleanse your body of toxins, and watch your allergies and your emotions.

Remedies

Cleansing Diet

Since toxins can raise systolic (and perhaps diastolic) pressure, a cleansing diet used for a few days may help. This could be a juice program, or a mono-diet, such as that recommended by Alan H. Nittler, M.D.[15] It consists of as much as you wish of one or two raw foods of your choice: grapes, grapefruit, or watermelon, celery, or whatever. The brown rice and natural, unsweetened fruit juice diet is also excellent when used for three days. Whatever the cleansing diet, not only are toxins eliminated, but your digestive apparatus is given a rest. The systolic pressure usually drops.

Garlic

One remedy which seems to benefit everyone is garlic!

You may have heard about garlic all of your life because in past years garlic was used to help many health problems. Garlic is now having a revival. It is being eaten fresh in salad dressings, on garlic bread, etc., or used in tablets with parsley included, and in garlic oil capsules. It has been found to help remove toxins, revitalize the blood, stimulate blood circulation, help make blood vessels more supple, and normalize intestinal flora. Maurice Mességué, the french herbal expert, states that garlic acts as a tonic, a vermifuge (kills worms or parasites), and is also a laxative, diuretic, antiseptic and antibacterial agent (a natural antibiotic). He adds "It not only stimulates vitality, but wherever I found healthy people, I found that they were garlic eaters."[16]

Harald J. Taub, former editor of *Prevention*, in an article, "Garlic Oil for Healthier Arteries," tells of a physician at the University of Geneva who tested garlic oil on a group of high blood pressure patients. After weeding out those with kidney dysfunction, he found that the administration of garlic relieved headaches and dizziness within five days.[16] *Lancet*, the English Medical journal, reported that garlic can also reduce cholesterol.[16]

A *Prevention* reader wrote, "After reading about taking garlic for healthier arteries, I decided to try garlic perles to lower my blood pressure. After taking garlic for about five weeks, it dropped from 140/90, where it had been for some time, (my doctor considered it on the high side of normal) to 126/90. Just to make sure, I had the clinic attendant take it a second time and it was the same. Now that the systolic pressure had dropped as a result of taking garlic, I am hoping my diastolic will also drop after a few more weeks."[16]

If garlic seems to cause gas or belching, persevere. It may merely indicate the vanquishing of your intestinal flora, as described in the chapter on indigestion. Also, if you don't wish to be socially ostracized because of garlicky breath, you can chew a few parsley leaves after eating the garlic, or take the garlic in tablet form or in perles, which tests have shown to be the equivalent of fresh garlic.[16] Taking two of these with your evening meal or at bedtime may solve your problem.

Alan H. Nittler, M.D., recommends fresh garlic cloves for lowering blood pressure. He believes a patient should find his own dosage. He can try one clove, or two, or three or four, adding them gradually until results are obtained. However, according to Harald J. Taub, in his article, "Garlic Oil for Healthier Arteries,"[16] garlic oil perles provide the same effect as fresh garlic. Garlic perles are small capsules, which contain garlic oil. Swallowed whole the taste and after-odor of garlic is avoided. Even better, take garlic plus parsley in tablet form.

One woman with a blood pressure reading of 200/100 reduced her blood pressure to 140/84 within *seven* days by taking extract of garlic, in deodorized perle form, available at health stores from a company well known for its natural supplements. Her dosage during this dramatic lowering procedure was 3 perles, three times daily. After the pressure had dropped, she then took, and still takes, one of these same perles three times daily, for maintenance purposes.

Cholesterol.

Does lecithin emulsify cholesterol in the body? Many doctors refuse to believe it. You can tell your doctor that in the *American Journal of Digestive Diseases*, April, 1952, two researchers reported that 122 patients were given foods extremely high in cholesterol, and instructed to add a teaspoon of soybean lecithin with each meal. Twenty-three patients, serving as controls, did not take the lecithin. Those who took it had a 79% decrease in cholesterol, whereas those who did not take it, did not experience a decrease.

Another example: Lester M. Morrison, M.D., reported in *Geriatrics* (Vol. 133, pages 12–19) that twenty-one of his patients had been given a low fat diet plus cholesterol reducing drugs, to no avail. He then told them to take two tablespoons of soy lecithin granules (available at health stores) three times daily. The results were dramatic. One woman had an unbelievably high cholesterol level of 1,012 (although normal levels vary, most physicians consider any reading higher than 200 questionable). This woman had been on a prolonged anticholesterol drug program and cholesterol-free diet, neither of which had affected her cholesterol. But soy lecithin lowered the high reading to 322 the first month, then to 186, or normal by the third month. Most of Dr. Morrison's patients were later able to maintain a normal cholesterol with only one or two tablespoons of lecithin granules daily. Soybean lecithin appears to work faster than egg yolk lecithin.

Doctors at Simon Stevin Research Institute, Bruges, Belgium, reported that 100 patients, given soybean lecithin for fourteen days, experienced a definite reduction in blood fat. (*Medical World News*, Nov. 22, 1974.)

High cholesterol is often accompanied by a high triglyceride level. Almost every nutritional nutrient is involved in stabilizing the cholesterol. Pectin is effective, as is a high protein diet, providing it does not contain fat. *Science News*, March, 1973, has stated that Vitamin C also flushes cholesterol out of arteries and body organs.

According to the new theory that the diastolic pressure reflects the atherosclerosis or artery plugging, usually due to deposits of cholesterol embedded in fat, [17] you now know what to do. Instead of avoiding the high cholesterol foods which are also highly nutritious foods, such as eggs, some organ meats, etc., nutritional physicians merely add lecithin granules or liquid to your diet. The granules can be sprinkled over salads, or added to juices. I have explained how liquid lecithin is used in my book, *Secrets of Health and Beauty*. [23] If you are confused about the saturated fat versus the unsaturated fat controversy, don't go overboard on either. Some *natural* saturated (animal) fat appears to be well used by the body.

Vitamin E can help. It is true that in patients with an elevated blood pressure, too much Vitamin E can cause a rise in blood pressure. Wilfrid E. Shute, M.D., says, "On the other hand, small doses of Vitamin E have been shown to decrease the peripheral resistance and lower blood pressure. Therefore, in such cases we are careful to control the blood pressure with the modern hypertensive drugs and usually begin treatment of such patients with a lower dosage of Vitamin E."[18]

The entire B complex and calcium have been generally recommended by nutritionists because these substances have a known calming and relaxing effect on nerves. Since high blood pressure can be caused by excessive contraction of the muscle walls of the arteries, *The Journal of the American Medical Association*[21] reported that because magnesium relaxed these muscles, it was also an effective treatment for hypertension.[26]

Allergies

Few people realize that allergies can raise the blood pressure suddenly and act as a stimulant. This rise usually appears in the systolic reading. Lloyd Rosenvold, M.D., a specialist in hypertension, observed a patient whose pressure shot up from normal to 230 systolic, approximately six hours after eating wheat.[9] Even some vitamins can act as allergens for some people. I know one person who cannot take Vitamin A in any supplement form—or bingo, up goes his pressure! Vitamin A in natural food or cod liver oil does not affect him adversely.

Others have trouble with milk, chocolate, orange juice and a host of others. Coffee raises the blood pressure of some people because of its stimulating effect. You will have to learn what affects *you*. For further help in identifying and treating allergies, see Chapter Three.

Meanwhile, once allergens have been completely eliminated, the effects usually disappear in several days.

Obesity

Obesity has been correlated with high blood pressure. A study of 800 Polynesians in the remote island of Pukapuka disclosed that the natives were almost completely free of high blood pressure, heart problems and diabetes. These natives are not overweight. They consume no alcohol, little sugar, no salt, bread, jam, tea, coffee or cake. They also eat an eighty percent intake of naturally saturated fat in the form of coconut oil. Yet they have the lowest pulse rate and the lowest cholesterol of any group ever studied.[25]

More frequent, smaller meals, have been found better for hypertensives than fewer large meals. In fact, the heavier the meal, the higher the blood pressure.[1]

Contaminants

How can you protect yourself against the present-day contaminants found to be a factor in high blood pressure, especially cadmium, a medically confirmed cause?

One way is to avoid smoking (tobacco smoke contains cadmium), but if you are a target of others who blow smoke your way, even though you are a nonsmoker, there is protection against cadmium (see Chapter 19), as well as nitrates and nitrites. According to Harald J. Taub, author of the book *Keeping Healthy in a Polluted World*,[26] tobacco has been found to constrict the arteries, thus raise blood pressure.[1] However, to give you some protection against these various contaminants you cannot control, Vitamin C helps to detoxify the effects on your body.[26]

Salt

There is a misunderstanding about salt. It is true that many studies show that those who eat a great deal of salt have higher blood pressure than those who do not. In fact, one report states that hypertensives eat four times as much salt as nonhypertensives. As a result, one physician states that if you are suffering from high blood pressure you should eat no more than one level teaspoon daily.[2] But herein lies a discrepancy. What *kind* of salt?

There are two general categories of salt: common table salt which appears on every grocery shelf in the world, and *whole* sea salt. There is a tremendous difference between the two, even though they taste the same.

Dr. Royal Lee stated (*Let's Live*, 1961) "When sea water dries up, the sodium chloride is the first to separate by crystallization. Rainfall aids in washing and draining away the other factors, leaving only sodium chloride. Sodium chloride is commonly used as a table salt."

Whole sea salt, on the other hand, is sea water carefully and naturally sundried so that other factors, called minerals (because they occur in small or trace amounts) are still present. According to research cited in an article from *Scientific American*, health requires astonishingly small amounts of these trace minerals. This salt, then, is *whole* salt, containing sodium chloride, but also approximately 15% in trace minerals, which are the health-giving elements and have been said to buffer and protect the body from too much sodium chloride. I, personally, refuse to buy or use common table salt for this reason. I have various analyses before me. Although they vary, one is of the most common brand found on grocery shelves and used by virtually most households in the world. It contains 99% sodium chloride, plus one part per million of some heavy metals such as lead.

The labels do not necessarily tell you the truth. One chemist told me that he had purchased a table salt at a supermarket, and a so-called "sea salt" from a health store. On analyzing them in the laboratory, he found them *both* containing nearly 100% sodium chloride. The manufacturer of some "sea salt" reasons that if the salt comes from the sea, as it probably did, it is "sea salt," not realizing (or not telling the truth) that the precious minerals were washed away during processing, leaving mainly sodium chloride. For this reason I will break my rule of not mentioning brand names. I buy Chico San salt, at health stores. It is a whole, naturally solar-dried salt imported from France. I am told that even this fine salt cannot tell the full story on its label, but can say "salt" only, not what kind.

There are also mined land salts. If they are whole salts, they are acceptable. Don't be afraid to eat some salt. The body needs it. Proof is evident in those who suffer from heat prostration after losing their supply of sodium through perspiration. Taking sodium restores that deficit. Fatigue can also be a symptom of sodium deficiency, which often can be corrected safely by taking a bit of the right kind of salt. Another need for sodium is in connection with the body's digestive hydrochloric acid which needs sodium for its manufacture. So salt-free diets can be dangerous. You can cut salt *down, but not out* using less salt, and substituting whole sea salt for sodium chloride. There are also herbal mixtures with a bit of salt added which can help solve your problem. Salt, like sugar and alcohol, are habit forming. Children do not like salt. Adults have increased it so that it becomes a habit.

Nothing makes a good cook, who prides herself on her season-ing, angrier than to see someone grab the salt shaker and pour it over a carefully seasoned food before even tasting it.

One way to avoid too much salt, is to use less in cooking, let-ting the individual add his own, after tasting. Watch out, too, for salted nuts, potato chips and corn chips, even popcorn, be-fore buying—all are salted with the usual high sodium chloride table salt. Being tasty, it is hard to stop eating these snacks. It would be better if you fixed your own, using whole sea salt in moderation. Sodium chloride salt has also been added to salted meats (ham, bacon, etc.), salted fish, and many canned foods. Even baby food is not immune. The reason is, that though chil-dren do not crave salt, the salt (and sugar too) is added for the parents who taste the food before offering it to their babies.

Edema

Edema, or fluid retention in the body, may be traced to too much salt, which tends to retain water, or to malfunctioning kidneys. You can usually tell if you have edema by looking at your ankles to see if they are swollen. The average doctor will immediately put you on a salt-free, or a low-salt diet. Or he will prescribe diuretics. There is a better way to handle edema. A healthy body should have not only sodium (only an excess of which tends to hold water), but potassium, another mineral, which releases the water from the body.

Adelle Davis has written, "High blood pressure has been pro-duced in animals merely by keeping them on a potassium-deficient diet, or by feeding them excessive amounts of salt which causes so much potassium to be lost in the urine that a deficiency results. In either case, so much water is retained that the volume of blood increases and the blood pressure is ele-vated."[17] Potassium can be taken in supplement form but accord-ing to Digestive Disease, April, 1973, p. 289, the supplements have caused gastric ulcers. It is preferable to take potassium in natural foods: green leafy vegetables, dried nuts and fruits, and tomato juice.

John M. Ellis, M.D. has done years of research with Vitamin B-6 which he has found controls *naturally* the sodium-potassium balance in the body (he recommends 50 mg. daily). Texas ranchers who are patients of Dr. Ellis have told him they could cinch their belts to the last notch by taking Vitamin B-6 without any other change in their diet.[20] Remember, when taking any single B vitamin, to add the entire B complex, to avoid imbalance of the B factors. Wheat germ, organic liver in some form, or brewer's yeast are rich sources of the entire B complex.

Dangers of Drug Diuretics

Now for those diuretics, sometimes called water pills. Brace yourself, because I get angry every time I think of them. Drug diuretics work so violently and so fast to rid the body of fluid, that the patient is usually knocked out after taking them.

At one "reducing farm" operated by a physician, attendees with edema (a common cause of overweight) were given a drug diuretic on arrival soon after their medical check-up. The patients spent the night going to the bathroom and several, whom I knew personally, lost an average of seven pounds each, in one night! They could scarcely move the next day, while the staff was congratulating them on becoming "so thin, already." Afterwards they were fed mainly on carrot sticks until they reached home, weak and emaciated and so ravenous they rushed to their refrigerators and gained back all their lost weight in two weeks flat. The diuretic drug action was not only a shock to the body, which likes gradual, not sudden changes, but more serious, with the great loss of fluids, they had also lost their supply of B vitamins (which are water soluble) and potassium, nutrients needed for health.

Another woman I have observed was suffering from edema, associated with a heart ailment. Twice, after the edema built up to a high level, her doctor gave her a drug diuretic. Each time she lost about fourteen pounds in approximately a week, and both times, lost her memory and her ability to think clearly. Each time it took months for her to regain mental normality, which she finally did on taking a high vitamin-mineral dosage on her own to compensate for the loss from the sudden, violent diuretic drug treatment.

There are safe, gentle herbal diuretics that work more slowly, but also more safely. These include a combination of herbs, as well as single herbs such as Buchu, Juniper, and many others at health stores. (Do not ask your health store operator to prescribe for you—she or he may land in jail.) Vitamin C and magnesium are also diuretics.

The homeopathic cell salt, Natrum Sulphate or phosphate of soda, abbreviated as *Nat. Sulph.*, also works naturally and safely when dissolved dry on the tongue. Cell salts are not a figment of the imagination as proved by a husband-wife team who were taking different cell salts for different conditions. Since they look and taste alike, one day the husband accidentally picked up his wife's *Nat. Sulph.* which she was taking for edema, thinking they were his own. Later in the day he said, "I cannot understand why I have been running to the bathroom all day." His wife answered, "So *that* is what happened to my cell salts which so mysteriously disappeared!"

Kidneys

Kidney dysfunction is usually associated with high blood pressure. The reason is that the heart pumps all the blood through the circulatory system every seven minutes, including the kidneys.[1] If the kidneys become clogged with uric acid and other deposits, toxins cannot be expelled properly, the blood is not properly purified, or edema may appear, and the blood pressure may become elevated. There are several ways out of this dilemma.

For years doctors have warned against protein, as a cause of kidney damage. More recent findings show just the opposite. Patients with kidney disease have been found to recover much more rapidly and kidney biopsies confirm this improvement when such patients take sufficient protein daily.[17]

Yet most orthodox doctors still believe that the kidney develops malfunction when people eat too much protein, particularly meat. One therapist, knowing that protein is highly necessary for body health, restricts only the red meats, which are believed to leave a greater residue of nitrogen. Animal proteins such as poultry, veal, lamb and some uncontaminated fish are allowed.

Another solution comes from the late D. C. Jarvis, M.D., who stated that it is not so much the added protein that creates a kidney problem, but the increased alkalinity of the blood produced by that protein. His recommendation was to offset the effect of added protein with acid in organic form: apple cider vinegar, apples, grapes, cranberries, or their juices. He recommended either four glasses of these juices daily, or a glass of water, with two teaspoons of apple cider vinegar four times daily, with, or between meals.[3]

He gave an example of the effect of this remedy for kidney dysfunction. In one case, a woman with pyelitis, an inflammation of the kidney which produces pus cells in the urine, had suffered from the condition for fifteen years. She began taking the apple cider vinegar in water and the condition disappeared for one year, at which time she discontinued the vinegar. The pyelitis reappeared, but again disappeared when she resumed the apple cider vinegar.

Adelle Davis reported that kidney disease was benefitted by Vitamin B-6, and lecithin. She added that calcification in kidneys is prevented by doubling the amount of calcium intake to offset a high phoshorus intake, found in protein. So when eating a high protein diet, be sure to add B-6, but also see if you need hydrochloric acid to help digest it, and avoid the toxins of undigested protein. The type of hydrochloric acid, as well as the dosage, is explained in my book, *Secrets of Health and Beauty*.[23] Or use apple cider vinegar as suggested by Dr. Jarvis. Protein *must* have acid for adequate digestion. (See chapter on indigestion.)

Cucumbers, fresh watermelon, or tea made from ground watermelon seeds, are considered good kidney cleansers, as is parsley. Parsley tea is made by simmering a bunch of parsley about the size of that found in grocery stores in water to cover, in which it is then allowed to cool. This can be sipped warm by the cupful, or cooled in the refrigerator and drunk slowly. Asparagus is also considered a good kidney cleanser. Perhaps the best of all is chamomile tea, which, as described under gall bladder, may dissolve gravel and other deposits. Chamomile tea is also calming and is often used as an aid for insomnia. Herbologists believe it should be continued a month after kidney symptoms cease. The old-time remedy, cranberry juice, is also helpful.

Adrenals

Some doctors believe that the adrenals, in connection with high blood pressure, are even more important to consider than the kidneys. No doubt both are involved. The adrenal glands lie perched atop the kidneys. As described before, they produce the fight-or-flight reaction when a person is faced with great stress. If this happens often, the adrenal overactivity may become chronic, and may contribute to high blood pressure. Presumably, this may be registered in the systolic pressure.

Remedies for overworked adrenals include pantothenic acid (a B vitamin), magnesium, calcium and Vitamin C. Of great importance, too, the adrenals are the body's reservoir for Vitamin C storage. If you have a shock such as an accident, a death in the family, even an upsetting argument with your husband, wife or children, the Vitamin C supply in your adrenals is used up in seconds. So Vitamin C should be taken regularly for preventive protection during such emergencies, and replaced immediately after they occur. The whole adrenocortical extract also relaxes overworked adrenals by temporarily supplying all needed hormones to allow the adrenal cortices to rest. This allows the blood pressure to drop.

Dr. Royal Lee believed that the kidneys function better if given a pure kidney tissue, called kidney cytotrophin. He also believed in support for the adrenals with a similar adrenal substance or cytotrophin. If the heart, or brain, or liver, were also showing stress, he supplied the cytotrophin for each organ or gland as needed.

These substances are available only from Standard Process Laboratories, Milwaukee, Wisc. 53201. They may be procured through a doctor *only*, whether an M.D., N.D., D.O., D.C. or D.D.S.

Other Glands

As stated earlier, Dr. M. E. Page finds that a well-adjusted body chemistry plus normal gland function helps a person to resist or prevent high blood pressure. But this resistance cannot be built upon feet of clay or a foundation of sand. Dr. Page insists that these glands need protein, all vitamins and minerals and a minimum of manmade carbohydrates such as white sugar, white flour, and other processed, devitalized foods. Otherwise the glands do not have the proper "fuel" needed to manufacture hormones to build and maintain body health.[14]

Digestants are often needed to digest protein. Papaya, peppermint tea and/or hydrochloric acid-Betaine, plus pepsin, have proved successful, presumably for the hydrochloric, but Guyon Richards, M.D., of England, says, "I have never failed with the use of pepsin (in elixir or liquid form) to get the blood pressure down. Both pepsin and pancreas have proved useful in treating high blood pressure. Every patient whose blood pressure was raised, I have found deficient in pepsin."[24]

Another glandular aid is a protein product which contains 100% glandular substances, including heart as well as many other valuable organ factors. This substance, designed to feed and nourish glands, contains no fillers and is desiccated and defatted at such low heat that all natural factors are carefully preserved. It is a high quality protein in powder or tablet form.

For information on the source of this product, write Corron Formulas, P.O. Box 1021, Pacific Palisades, Calif. 90272.

Strokes

To protect yourself against strokes, it is not only necessary to lower your blood pressure, but also to strengthen the walls of the capillaries through which the blood flows and where a bursting point may occur. Fragile capillaries have been strengthened by sufficient protein, Vitamin E, lecithin or choline (a B vitamin) pantothenic acid (another B vitamin) ascorbic acid for Vitamin C as well as the Vitamin C complex known as the bioflavonoids which contain, among other factors, rutin, especially potent for capillary strength.[17]

Avoid the Pill! A study involving the research of doctors of 91 hospitals in 12 cities showed that the birth control pill alone can increase the chance of a stroke. (*Journal of the American Medical Association*, Feb. 17, 1975).

Dr. Evan Shute states that Vitamin E offers protection against strokes and clots.[27]

One of the homeopathic cell salts, *Kali. Mur.* (potassium chloride) has been used with success for dissolving clots. The clot dissolution is accomplished without excessive thinning of blood, which drugs may produce, and without the danger of internal bleeding. If this remedy is begun within a few hours after a stroke, rapid and complete recovery has been obtained in numerous cases.

Alcohol

Some doctors have long told patients that a little alcohol will dilate their arteries. But note that word, "little"! A study conducted by three doctors revealed that though alcohol may relieve pressure and pains in angina, its value is due to a sedative action, not to dilation of arteries. The researchers learned that alcohol can create a false feeling of fitness and security which may lead to fatal consequences. Perhaps an occasional beer or a small glass of wine may help relaxation, but many do not stop with one. Alcohol also steals B vitamins from the body, and B vitamins protect your nerves. So don't kid yourself. There are safer tranquilizers that don't lead to great danger.[28]

William A. Brams, M.D. states, "Blood pressure is increased during intercourse, but the rise is of short duration and generally does not induce harmful effects *in the absence of complicating conditions*. Undue shortness of breath, tightness, pain in the chest or excessive fatigue after the exertion are signs that the strain has been too great . . . abstinence is recommended if any of these symptoms develop. Your doctor may advise you to abstain until your blood pressure has been reduced and the symptoms have been brought under control."[29]

Exercise

If your high blood pressure persists, doctors may suggest that you change your life style. Lose weight, cut smoking down or out, relax (discussed later) and increase your physical activity, including gentle exercise. Many doctors agree that there should be no violent sports and that jogging can actually be dangerous in cardiovascular cases.[30] Lloyd Rosenvold, M.D., believes that a brisk ½-mile walk is safer and helps circulation. Such exercise tones up the blood vessel network, he says, and helps to normalize minor blood pressure elevation.[9]

A nutritional consultant agrees. She says any exercises which involve the body *above the waist* should be minimal. If you do neck or head-bending exercises, do them gently without tension, she suggests.

Dr. Norman N. Kaplan[2] believes that isotonic exercise, which involves muscular activity, is beneficial. This includes swimming, bicycling, rowing, running (not jogging) and rhythmic calisthenics. Such exercise brings fresh oxygen to the muscles, and although, according to Dr. Kaplan, the heart pumps more blood and the heart rate increases, the blood pressure changes very little.

On the other hand, Dr. Kaplan does not recommend isometric exercise. This type of exercise involves lifting, pushing heavy weights, and tightening muscles while braced against fixed objects. In this case, he states that the heart rate does not increase much, but the blood pressure does, due to tensing muscles which tighten blood vessels and increase the pumping action of the heart.

However, there is another side of this isometric story. Two New York researchers report that only eighteen seconds of isometric exercise daily are amazingly effective in controlling high blood pressure. They placed fifteen hypertensive subjects on this exercise regimen, for five to eight weeks. All showed a marked decrease of both systolic and diastolic pressure, even though no drugs were given. No side effects of the exercise were noted. The subjects, for the most part, reported a feeling of fitness, better posture and a decrease of pendulous flesh. The two researchers who made this discovery were Broino Kiveloff, M.D., Chief Psychiatrist in the Department of Physical Medicine and Rehabilitation of the New York Infirmary, and Olive Huber, Ph.D., Professor Emeritus of the Department of Physiology and Health, Hunter College.[31]

The exercise can be done at home. It is as follows; Stand, relaxed, with your knees and elbows just slightly flexed. Contract every muscle of your body five or six seconds, while you count six slow counts *and while you simultaneously breathe* in and out. Repeat this three times daily.

Drs. Kiveloff and Huber theorize that the benefit of this exercise may be due to the fact that the arterial blood supply to the capillaries is being increased without blocking the return blood flow in the veins through undue strain or mechanical resistance. The sympathetic nervous system may also be helped.

If you are in any doubt about the effect of this exercise on you, check with your doctor.

Dr. Kaplan warns against strenuous weekend exercise which, after days, weeks or months of inactivity, may be hazardous. However, he reports studies in which a regular program of fifteen minutes of calisthenics daily, swimming two hours a week, or playing volleyball have helped reduce blood pressure in mild hypertensives. He sums up, "A gradually accelerating course of exercise may help lower your blood pressure." Golf may be an asset provided you stop before you get too tired, even if you have not completed the nine or eighteen holes you had planned. Tennis, more strenuous, should be checked with your doctor.

Emotions and Nervous Tension

Emotional stress is well accepted as a factor in high blood pressure. There are at least two logical reasons. Tension constricts the entire body, including the arteries and capillaries, which in turn restrict blood flow. But stress and tension also affect the adrenals, setting off an entire chain of physiological reactions. This is not merely guess work. Hans Selye, M.D., the internationally respected expert on stress, has proved the concept, and photographs in color show what happens to all organs of the body when subjected to prolonged or continued stress. The organs, as shown in photographs (which I have seen), when subjected to stress become engorged and congested beyond recognition or belief.

Everyone is subjected to stress these days. It is impossible to dodge or run away from it. So what can you do? The first thing you must *not* do, when you realize you are tense, or when your doctor tells you your blood pressure is high, is to grit your teeth and clench your fists and say, "I *must* relax." This attitude merely makes you more tense and defeats your goal. Here are better suggestions by doctors and tension experts to help you: [29,32]

1. Change your life style to increase physical activity and more relaxation.

2. Take a nap, a siesta, or "that pause that refreshes," several times daily.

3. Don't push or drive yourself. Learn to enjoy life and flow with it, not push against it. *Let down and let go* whenever possible.

4. Do work which is suitable for you. If you can't change your job, change yourself and your attitude toward it. Cultivate a calm mind, a tranquil outlook. Toward things that bug you take a "so what?" or a mañana point of view.

5. Balance your work with play.

6. Do not, I repeat *not*, become a drug or tranquillizer addict. This does not solve anything in the long run except to create still more problems. Don't become an alcoholic, either. Instead, take calcium, B vitamins, magnesium—all calmers. Try the

homeopathic tranquillizers which are safe and nonhabit-forming. One, called *Nerve Tonic,* consists of several Schuessler cell salts which are soothing minerals in tiny sweet pellets. These are dissolved dry on the tongue and not washed down with water. Before a trip to the dentist or some other stressful situation you may dread, they are wonderful.

Another version is called *Calms Forté.* These are larger tablets to be used according to the label. They are the same homeopathic cell salts fortified with soothing herbs, including chamomile. They are used as a relaxant, or for insomnia, have no side effects, are not habit forming and are absolutely harmless. They are found in homeopathic pharmacies and some health stores. Because they do not leave you with a hangover and do aid nervous tension and sleeplessness, they are becoming extremely popular. They contain no drugs.

7. If you are seething with resentment, take a warm bath to relax, or work or walk it off, or blow off steam to a patient friend or counselor. Don't let it pile up until you explode. Strokes have been caused by such action. If a person irritates you, mentally bless instead of damning him. You will find it a potent steam reliever.

8. Science has recently learned that oxygen is rejuvenating, improves memory and lowers blood pressure. Don't allow yourself to become a shallow breather or a nonbreather. Watch yourself as you work to see if you tense up and forget to breathe. You can also get more oxygen into your body by taking the right amount of Vitamin E for you (see Chapter 19 on Heart Problems) and Vitamin C, both of which provide oxygen to your body. Or you can do *deep breathing* whenever you feel yourself becoming tense. Let your entire rib cage or diaphragm expand sideways as you fill it, as well as your upper and lower lungs, with air. Speakers and singers and actors and actresses who feel jittery before a public appearance have learned this trick of deep breathing for a few seconds until their nerves become steady.

Leslie O. Korth, D.O. of England, believes that one activating cause of high blood pressure is shallow, ineffective breathing.

He says that not only has hypertension been normalized by correct breathing in three to six weeks by his patients, but shortness of breath, insomnia, irritability, head and chest pressure, headache, palpitation, giddiness, and poor memory have been corrected or improved. He found that of one hundred professional singers (who breathe correctly) not a single one suffered from high blood pressure! He states that his method of breathing will not only bring down high blood pressure but will also revitalize the entire nervous system and the whole organism, as well as improve digestion if the exercises are practiced immediately after meals. He contends that most people do too much inhaling, if they remember to breathe at all, and not enough exhaling. Here is the method:

"Inhale slowly through the nose, allowing the lower abdomen to protrude slightly. At the same time lift your ribs upward and outward in order to fill *all* lung space *completely* with air. Don't strain. Easy does it.

"Now, for the most import part: Exhale through the mouth, on a sustained note of "O," and exhaling slowly *to the last possible second*, though without strain. You can make a sound if you wish, or exhale quietly. Your lips will give the impression to others that you are whistling.

"Do this three times daily for 10 minutes at each practice. Do it while sitting, standing, after eating, before bedtime or while walking upstairs or on the level."[33]

9. If you are a deadline hater, rearrange your way of life. Do not put things off until the last moment so that you blow if the car in front of you seems too slow, or the people around you uncooperative. There is no need for the photofinish. Do things ahead of time, plan ahead, and arrive with that delicious and luxurious feeling of being ready before you need to be. It will take years off your face and points off your blood pressure.

10. If you find yourself becoming tense, or if you are too tense to sleep when You go to bed, try the rag doll technique. Relax each foot until they both feel heavy. Then proceed upward to your ankles, your knees, thighs, buttocks, abdomen,

arms, back, chest, back of the neck, face, eyes and scalp. Especially drop your shoulders. This complete "letting go" is beneficial to ciruclation nerves and blood pressure.

11. Try prayer. Shift your burden to a higher power, then forget about it. Miracles often happen when you do.

Dr. Herbert Benson, an associate professor of medicine at Harvard, and cardiologist at Beth Israel Hospital in Boston, stated that meditation lowers heart rate, blood pressure and metabolism so effectively that he now teaches the exercise to add to any other treatment that may prove useful. Here is his exercise: Sit up straight. Let all your muscles go limp. Close your eyes and think about your breathing. As you exhale, say some short, meaningless word such as "one." Ignore all extraneous thoughts.

Dr. Benson found that this simple exercise practised by forty patients with moderate to higher blood pressure, repeated twice daily for twenty minutes at a time, produced a significant lowering of blood pressure in all but two patients. It also improved the patients' sense of well-being and ability to cope with the world around them.

Emergency and Other Remedies

If your pressure has risen to a frightening high, there are two emergency remedies you can resort to. One is a clear water enema, as suggested by Lloyd Rosenvold, M.D.[31] He states that he has witnessed in his patients a drop of 40 points in the systolic pressure and 20 points in the diastolic within an hour after a clear water enema. "This drop was maintained for several hours," he reported.

A doctor gave me this emergency remedy. He has found the fastest way to reduce blood pressure is by the use of colonic irrigations. His method: A colonic—one, daily, for three days. Then two a week for four weeks. Then once a month. In one of his cases the pressure was too high to register. After the first colonic, the pressure dropped to 300/260. Continuing the colonics, by the second day, sixteen hours later, the alarming pressure had dropped to 145/80.

I have known people who experienced an immediate drop in blood pressure following a chiropractic or osteopathic adjustment in the atlas-axis area of the spine.

Dr. F. M. Houston, in his excellent do-it-yourself book on acupressure *(Acupuncture Without Needles)*, states that he has found one method which brings blood pressure down faster than any other he has ever witnessed. He describes how it is done: "Put your index fingers straight into your ears. Press firmly then lift slightly forward toward the nose. Hold this contact for several minutes. The blood pressure may be reduced at the first treatment.[34]

A Surprise Remedy

I have chanced upon a surprising remedy for high blood pressure, as found by two physicians in a California State Prison. The subjects, inmates of the prison, were elderly, hypertensives, did not drink alcohol, did eat prison food, and at the time of the study (1932–3) were subjected to no physical strain and very little mental strain. Yet their blood pressure was high, their average systolic reading 180.

The men were given a rounded tablespoon of powdered whey, dissolved in water, three times a day. Treated with no other medication or remedy than the whey, within three months, the systolic pressure dropped from 180 to 148. A second group was tested. These men were engaged in active employment and their systolic pressure averaged 194. On the whey treatment the pressure dropped within five days to 171, and within twenty days to 163.[35]

The explanation given was that the whey completely changed the intestinal flora for the better, acted as a mild laxative, and may have aided in detoxification. Powdered whey is a derivative of milk and is available at health stores.

A Testimonial

I received a letter which tells a success story of a woman who brought down her own blood pressure by natural methods. She is a "store hostess" in a well-known and respected natural organic farm health foods store. She wrote, "Nutrition has been a great help to me personally since I have had high blood sugar, blood clots with attendant higher blood pressure, which I identified as due to atherosclerosis, much to my orthodox doctor's unhappy surprise (he does not believe in nutrition). He was even unhappier when I brought my blood pressure down from 146 to 117 (systolic) with Vitamin E, soy oil and lecithin over a period of two weeks. He refused to believe it and checked several times. He, of course, was taught that only drugs could have any effect on blood pressure."

Homeopathy can often prove miraculous. One homeopathic M.D. finds that the blood pressure rises if the hypothalamus gland is malfunctioning. This can be brought to normal, according to this doctor, by the homeopathic substance, *gelsemium*. In some cases, however, if the kidneys are at fault, this doctor uses the homeopathic substance *Renin*. The results have been spectacular. (For information on locating a homeopathic physician in your area, write National Center for Homeopathy, Suite 506, 6231 Leesburg Pike, Falls Church, Virginia, 22044.)

So consider the suggestions discussed in this chapter and work out your own plan to cope with your high blood pressure naturally and permanently.

REFERENCES
(See *Bibliography* for fuller details.)

1. *High Blood Pressure*. A composite report of experts, Science of Life Books Pty. Ltd., 4–12 Tattersalls Lane, Melbourne, Victoria 3000, Australia.
2. Norman M. Kaplan, *Your Blood Pressure: The Most Deadly High*.
3. D.C. Jarvis, M.D., *Folk Medicine*.
4. Bernard Jensen, D.C., N.D., *The Science and Practice of Iridology*.
5. *M.D.*, March, 1973; also *Medical World News*, Dec. 1, 1972.
6. Edwin Wood, M.D., Professor of Medicine, University of Pennsylvania, "Modern Concept of Cardiovascular Disease," August, 1972.

7. *Lancet*, January 20, 1973.
8. Harald J. Taub, *Keeping Healthy in a Polluted World*. See also: Henry A. Schroeder, M.D., *The Trace Elements and Man*; Ruth Adams and Frank Murray, *Minerals, Kill or Cure?*
9. Lloyd Rosenvold, M.D., *Drop Your Blood Pressure*.
10. *JAMA*, October 25, 1971; *Lancet*, December 16, 1972.
11. *JAMA*, September 10, 1972.
12. Arthur F. Coca, M.D., *The Pulse Test*.
13. Linda Clark, *Get Well Naturally*, p. 205.
14. Melvin E. Page, D.D.S., *Degeneration to Regeneration*.
15. Alan H. Nittler, *A New Breed of Doctor*.
16. *Natural Health World*. July, 1974; *Lancet*, December 29, 1973; Mailbag, *Prevention*, p. 182, October, 1974. See also: Maurice Mességué, *Way to Natural Health and Beauty*; Harald J. Taub, "Garlic Oil for Healthier Arteries, *Prevention*, April, 1974.
17. Adelle Davis, *Let's Get Well*.
18. Wilfrid E. Shute, with Harald J. Taub, *Vitamin E for Ailing and Healthy Hearts*.
19. *Prevention*, page 222, July, 1973.
20. John M. Ellis, M.D., and James Presley, *Vitamin B-6, The Doctor's Report*.
21. *Journal of the American Medical Association*, February 22, 1965. See also: *American Heart Journal*, 1969; *American Journal of Clinical Nutrition*, June, 1964.
22. Melvin E. Page, D.D.S., *Anthropometrics*, July, 1964.
23. Linda Clark, *Secrets of Health and Beauty*.
24. Guyon Richards, M.D., *The Chain of Life*.
25. *San Francisco Chronicle*, February 6, 1970.
26. Harald J. Taub, *Keeping Healthy in a Polluted World*.
27. *Summary*, December, 1974.
28. *Jouranl of the American Medical Association*, May 27, 1950. See also: Linda Clark, *Get Well Naturally*.
29. William A. Brams, M.D., *How to Live With Your Blood Pressure*.
30. *Modern Medicine*, January 26, 1971.
31. *Rodale's Health Bulletin*, January 25, 1972.
32. Fred Kerner, *Dr. Hans Selye's Famous Concept of Stress and Your Heart*.
33. Leslie O. Korth, D.O., M.R.O., *Some Unusual Healing Methods*.

21: HYPOGLYCEMIA

(Low Blood Sugar)

Of all the ailments included in this book, hypoglycemia is perhaps the most common. Nearly everyone has it, and few realize it. Some have it in serious form; others in lighter degree. This is one disturbance which can be controlled by diet, but first it must be recognized. In general, it is a disease of civilization: refined foods, sugars and sugary foods, as well as excessive use of soft drinks, cola drinks, and coffee can lead it right to your door.

I am going to devote very little space to this disturbance, not because it is not important: it is *crucial*, but because there is so much information already available about it; what it is, and what to do about it. Fortunately it is a do-it-yourself treatment disease. Once you recognize the symptoms, and it has been diagnosed, nobody can pull you out except you, yourself.

In general, the symptoms are legion. Almost *any* symptom may be caused by hypoglycemia (or hyperinsulinism). It can cause intense irritability, shakiness, blackouts; it can mimic asthma, allergies, coronary thrombosis (heart attacks), epileptic seizures, psychomotor attacks, peptic ulcer or arthritis: you name it, it may be hypoglycemia in disguise.

Many doctors are self-styled experts on hypoglycemia, but really have not studied it in depth or understood it fully. Usually when you go to a doctor for any one of the above or a myriad of other complaints, an average doctor will put you through your paces and find nothing. So he tells you to seek psychiatric care, meaning that he considers it "all in your mind." This is where you must rebel. Since hypoglycemia *can* be diagnosed, run, don't walk to the nearest *specialist*. There are people in institutions who have been committed for no other reason than the fact that they are hypoglycemics and no one recognized it. Yet, had they known their condition, they could have stayed at home, followed the diet and remained well.

One food which acts as a deadly poison to hypoglycemics is sugar in any form! Yet there are doctors who actually prescribe a candy bar when you feel tired and shaky (symptoms of low blood sugar) on the mistaken belief that a sweet will elevate your blood sugar and make you feel better. It will—temporarily—but soon afterward your blood sugar will plummet even lower than it was originally, and you are now on an on-again, off-again merry-go-round, resulting in a malfunctiong pancreas which, believe me, can lead to trouble.

On the other hand, a hypoglycemia specialist who understands the disturbance will refer you to a medical laboratory for a five-hour, seven-specimen glucose tolerance test. Anything less than this, according to Dr. Alan H. Nittler, one of these specialists, is guesswork. This test will establish the exact status of your complaint, so that dietary management can then be begun to pull you out, and keep you out, of trouble.

In general, the diet is one that favors proteins, fresh vegetables and fruits, but *no man made sugar products:* candy, cakes, cookies, sweet beverages, etc. Even coffee can be a hazard. And once a hypoglycemic, you may always be prone to the trouble, even though you have eaten your way to apparent normalcy. For example, one woman who had given up coffee because, like sugar, it triggered her pancreas problem, decided (after months of feeling wonderful as a result of following the entire diet —really generous and easy to take), to reward herself with just one cup of coffee. The whole set of symptoms were back upon her without warning.

There are many books which tell you more about hypoglycemia and how to handle it. I will list just a few. I urge you to consult them.

1. The "bible": *Body, Mind and Sugar*, by E. M. Abrahamson, M.D. and A. W. Pezet.

2. *A New Breed of Doctor* by Alan H. Nittler, M.D.

3. *Low Blood Sugar and You* by Carlton Fredericks, Ph.D. and Herman Goodman, M.D.

4. *My Battle with Low Blood Sugar*, by G. M. Thienell, published by Exposition Press, 50 Jericho Turnpike, Jericho, N.Y. 11753. This is a charming short authobiography of a woman's struggle against low blood sugar. If you are hypoglycemic, you will find yourself on every page.

Except for No. 4, most of these books are in paperback, and are available at health stores. Or your local book store can probably locate them for you.

22: LEG CRAMPS

Many people panic because of leg cramps. Some seek the services of an orthodox doctor who may not realize that the problem has a simple cause, and may prescribe drugs which do not reverse the condition permanently. Actually, leg cramps have been found in thousands of people merely to be a deficiency of a nutrient which, when restored sufficiently, banishes the cramps forever. Leg cramps have been found to be due to a deficiency of the following:

1. Calcium (the most common)
2. Vitamin B-6 (as established by John M. Ellis, M.D.)
3. Vitamin E (to improve circulation).
4. Vegetable oils.

Peculiarly, these leg cramps usually attack during the night. They may be excruciatingly painful, occurring either in the calf of the leg, or in the foot. Since the deficiency cannot be corrected instantly, there are some relief measures you can use before you start your supplementation, come the light of day.

Turn over in bed on your back. Point your toes toward the

ceiling. This position will probably break the clutch of the cramp so that you can get back to sleep. If not, get up and walk around. If that doesn't help, get into a tub of warm-hot water until the cramping subsides.

Even during the daytime, a hand cramp, or a finger cramp may appear. Sometimes a cramp will catch you in the intercostal muscles, horizontally below your breastbone, causing you to believe it is a heart attack. It is not. It may occur as you lean over, forward, but still is nothing more than a calcium deficiency.

What kind of calcium should you take to prevent such cramps? Different calciums do different jobs in our body. Where bone meal is good for bones and a preventive for fractures, particularly in old people, other calciums such as calcium lactate help tissues and nerves and are quickly absorbed. Within a day or so after your cramp-warning that you are short in calcium, you should begin to see results. Calcium is also a natural tranquilizer and, according to Adelle Davis, the tablets (available from health stores) are "lullaby" pills. Taking some at bedtime or keeping them on your bedside table, in *addition* to incorporating extra calcium in your diet, is a good and harmless precaution.

Many patients are told, as they age, that they must not take calcium, since it piles up in the system and causes arthritis. The so called "piling up" is not caused by the calcium, which is more needed than ever as one ages, but by its lack of assimilation. Acid is needed in the body to dissolve the calcium so that it will *not* pile up in the joints. This acid may be Vitamin C, hydrochloric acid or apple cider vinegar taken in water. Dr. Jarvis, of Vermont fame, found that cattle fed apple cider vinegar, did not have calcium deposits, whereas those who were not fed the vinegar ration daily, did. Vitamin D, either in supplement form, or sensible exposure to sun, also helps calcium assimilation.

I cannot give you the dosage of any of these nutrients since I am not a doctor, but even if I were, I would not know. Each person differs from the next and you will have to find out what works for you.

Some people take the mineral *silica* which, it has been stated, changes into calcium in the body. Another quickly utilized calcium is the Schuessler cell salt, *Calc. Phos.* (Calcium Phosphorus). These tiny pellets are dissolved dry on the tongue. They are available both from homeopathic pharmacies and many health stores. Watch out for cow's milk. Though high in calcium, many are allergic to it.

Some people develop leg cramps after years of immunity. The reason may be that they are taking more protein in some form, or have added lecithin to their diet. Protein, even brewer's yeast, and lecithin, all excellent products, are high in phosphorus. Phosphorus is closely associated with calcium, and when it is excreted from the body it takes the calcium with it, leaving a deficiency in its wake. The solution to the problem is simple: take additional calcium to make up for the phosphorus-caused calcium loss.

One type of foot cramp, or a "Charley Horse," is due to lack of Vitamin B-6. Even stalwart men have been known to cry from the pain until they learned of and started taking B-6 on a regular basis. This type of cramp stopped abruptly. Dr. Ellis gave his patients never less than 50 mg. of B-6 daily for years without side effects, although when taking any single B vitamin, as we have noted, the whole family or complex should accompany it. This may be in the form of high vitamin B complex foods: brewer's yeast, liver, wheat germ, etc., or in supplement form. The reason: too much of one B vitamin may cause an imbalance in the others. Recently it has been discovered that when a higher protein diet is implemented, B-6 is also needed.

Vitamin E helps circulation in the legs (also cold feet), and when you find the right amount for you, that is your dosage. The Drs. Shute believe that the average person can take a minimum of 300 I.U. of Vitamin E daily. Others may or may not need more. Most nutritionists recommend 600-800 I.U. for men and 300-400 for women, first working up to these amounts.

Leg cramps in some cases have responded to adding vegetable oils to the diet. So if one element does not work, try another, or several. It is not necessary to be a victim of leg cramps.

23: THE NEUROMUSCULAR DISEASES:

Multiple Sclerosis, Muscular Dystrophy, Myasthenia Gravis

These three disturbances combine problems of nerve and muscle. Although many orthodox practitioners believe there is little or no help for these afflictions, if the tissues involved are still active and alive, though feeble, there is hope for recovery. These disorders are related in that there is wasting, weakness and loss of muscular control. Only if degeneration is too advanced, may complete paralysis result. Most orthodox practitioners are pessimistic because they are looking for a method of *drug control*, which has not come to light, at least for permanent help. They have overlooked the fact that nutrition not only *can* help, it *has* helped many recover from these disturbances. If you have, or a member of your family has, one of these afflictions, here are factors which, used in combination, have brought about definite improvement.

1. Natural unrefined foods, as many raw as possible, are a must.

2. Minerals are necessary: potassium to encourage muscle contraction; calcium for nerves; magnesium for muscle relaxation; manganese for muscle strengthening; and sodium for muscle stimulation.

3. Vitamins B complex for nerves, E for circulation and muscle strength.

4. Foods including protein (to build muscles) lecithin and vegetables oils for nerves and other functions. Fat has been found absolutely necessary to protect the myelin sheath, which, in turn, insulates nerves.

5. Exercise, rest, deep breathing, and a mild climate seem to encourage muscle repair. Peace of mind, even prayer, are valuable. If depression or other emotional reactions get out of hand, Vitamin C should be used liberally. This is because any emotional disturbance depletes the adrenal glands of their storage of Vitamin C within seconds, and this vitamin helps to protect the body from infections.

In addition to these general considerations, let's look at the specific measures recommended for these disturbances, separately.

Multiple Sclerosis

Early symptoms of MS, a disturbance of the central nervous system in league with weakened muscle reactions, include weakness, heaviness in the legs, brain dysfunction, numbness and tingling of the fingers and toes, visual disturbances (seeing double), bladder malfunction, giddiness, and a loss of balance. *But MS can also be misdiagnosed!* So if you have one or more of these symptoms, do not jump to false conclusions.

One deficiency in MS patients is a lack of unsaturated fatty acids, found in vegetable oils.[1] Roy L. Swanks, M.D., Ph.D. of the University of Oregon Medical School combined vegetable oils with cod liver oil (5 gms. of each daily) and if the treatment was started early, improvement occurred. As stated earlier, the reason for such treatment is that MS patients apparently need this fat-like substance for nerve insulation.

But the Vitamin B complex, and minerals suggested at the beginning of this chapter, as well as a great emphasis on raw foods, are also factors needed by the MS patient. Ebba Waerland, of Switzerland, advocates a program for MS which includes a short detoxifying program, followed by largely raw, unprocessed foods, no sugar, plenty of Vitamin B plus brewer's yeast. One of her patients who had suffered from MS for over a year recovered in three weeks.

However, the most famous treatment of MS in the world, is that of Dr. Joseph Evers, who has a clinic in Hachen, Westfallen, KR Arnesburg, West Germany. Thousands of MS patients have recovered on the Evers diet within a month, and have returned home to lead a normal life.

One patient, a minister in the U.S., was unable to walk when he began the Evers treatment at home. His recovery was so rewarding that he eventually hiked nine miles daily.

Here is the Evers diet, *which contains no denatured foods:*

Allowed foods

1. Raw milk and milk products, providing you are not allergic to them. If cow's milk upsets you, goat's milk may be substituted. Use butter, cheese and soured milks.

2. Sprouted grains such as rye and wheat.

3. All fruits, preferably fresh and raw.

4. Unprocessed honey.

5. Nuts and other oil-containing foods.

6. Organically grown *root* vegetables, particularly beets.

7. A raw egg daily (can be beaten into milk with honey as an eggnog).

Prohibited foods

1. Vegetable leaves and stems. Potatoes.

2. All fried, cooked, baked foods except whole grain, sour dough bread (see recipe).

3. Coffee, tea, cocoa, alcohol, mustard, salt, sugar or sugar substitutes.

Evers Home-made Sour Dough Rye Bread.
Use rye or wheat flour, or both combined. Add water, enough to knead well. Place in a bowl, cover with a cloth and let stand at room temperature until dough is slightly soured (overnight or a little longer). Bake at low temperature for four hours. Wait twenty-four hours before serving. It may crumble due to no yeast. Serve with pure butter.

There is one other European approach to MS devised by Roger MacDougal, of England, who recovered from MS. after twenty years and diagnoses by several physicians, including an internationally famous neurologist. Laboratory tests of brain and other tissues confirmed this diagnosis, yet Mr. MacDougal not only improved, at age sixty-two he recovered completely! He devised his own method which he has shared with thousands of other MS victims, who also recovered. Some were completely immobilized. Others were in wheelchairs.

Roger MacDougal also used diet to bring about his recovery. In some instances his diet is similar to the Evers' diet. In others it is just the opposite. Here is his routine:

No refined foods, white sugar, etc.

Vegetable oils, low animal fat intake.

High doses of a vitamin-mineral supplement plus vitamin B-12, given separately.

Chicken, fish, lean beef and lamb, plus emphasis on glandular meats: liver, kidney, tongue, sweetbreads and brain (all rich in vitamins and minerals).

All vegetables, including raw salads and potatoes!

The one major point of disagreement between the Evers and MacDougal diets is that MacDougal insists that there be a *complete* absence of foods containing gluten, whether they are from rye, wheat barley or oats. Those who used the MacDougal diet swear that their recovery began when they gave up gluten.

Since thousands have recovered on both diets, you can take your pick.

In this country, Carlton Fredericks, Ph.D., a nutrition researcher, suggests the use of six teaspoons daily of cold pressed wheat germ oil, either 8:1 or 10:1 ratio. This is available at health stores (or they can order) and is extremely expensive, but Dr. Fredericks finds it a powerful muscle stimulator which gets many a neuromuscular patient on his feet.

One surprising cause of MS has recently come to the attention of doctors. This is lead poisoning. A beautiful young dancer in Las Vegas contracted MS and was obliged to give up her career though she was only about thirty. She eventually was confined to a wheelchair, due to an inability to use her legs, and with a prognosis of a hopeless future. An alert doctor to whom she went, took a hair analysis and found her loaded with lead. She was put on lead-removing medication, plus minerals in which she was deficient, and she was also given ordinary baked beans daily (found by John J. Miller, Ph.D., to contain a lead-removing substance). She recovered in one year, resumed her career and began a crusade to encourage all MS victims to have a hair analysis.

The fact that this previous victim was in her thirties is not surprising. The average age for contracting the ailment seems to be between ages 20–40. Another pattern observable in MS is that the closer people live to the equator, the fewer cases of MS have been found. Dr. Paul Goldberg, a research scientist in Cambridge, Mass. has translated this statistic into a theory: that the closer to the equator, the more exposure to the sun (free of blocking contaminants, smog, etc.), the more Vitamin D is absorbed. Obviously not everyone can move toward the equator, but according to the Goldberg theory, what everyone can do is to take more calcium and Vitamin D in dietary supplements, either to prevent the disease, or arrest it in its earliest stages.[2]

One final observation. MS patients have been found to be deficient in linoleic acid. Researchers in England and Ireland have suggested taking two tablespoons of sunflower seed oil twice daily. A study of MS patients revealed that this therapy reduced the frequency of relapses following improvement in the MS itself.[3]

Sort out the information in this chapter used by others for

controlling MS, and work out your own program which is the near-equivalent of that provided in a European Spa. You can do it in your own home.

Myasthenia Gravis

MG is mainly a disease characterized by muscle weakness. Symptoms include fatigue, drooping eyelids, double vision, slurred speech, with trouble in chewing, swallowing and chest breathing, and in general, exhaustion of the voluntary muscles.

Adelle Davis has made the comforting statement, "If the diet is completely adequate, such rapid and astonishing improvement so frequently follows that there seems little justification for the belief that nothing can be done for myasthenia gravis." In fact, Adelle has enumerated examples of complete remission from this disease by dietary management. One woman who had had the ailment for twenty-seven years recovered.[4] Others also led normal lives once again.

In addition to a completely adequate diet, Adelle has advocated yeast, liver, eggs, Vitamin E and 50 mg. of manganese with each meal daily. Both Vitamin E and manganese are muscle strengtheners.

Dr. Emanuel Josephson was also reported, in *Prevention*, May 1973, as stating that myasthenia gravis patients, who, in addition to an adequate diet, took 50 mg. of manganese three times daily, one at each meal, recovered completely within several weeks.

Carlton Fredericks, Ph.D. recommends 750 mg. of pantothenic acid and 1,000 mg. of choline daily. Both are B vitamins. He also recommends B-6 as well as liver and yeast.

Others note the good effects of concentrated wheat germ oil, as suggested for MS.[5]

I have included in my book, *Secrets of Health and Beauty*, the case of a man afflicted with myasthenia gravis whose handshakiness was reversed within six weeks by taking liquid lecithin. Another victim was confined to a wheelchair. After two months on liquid lecithin he could raise his arms. After six months he could walk to the church altar to take communion. Today he plays golf. MG cases have been found to be deficient in lecithin. These cases just mentioned, achieved their improvement by taking one teaspoon of liquid lecithin morning and night.

MG patients have trouble swallowing hot drinks, but Belgian medical researchers found that cold drinks and ice cream were swallowed with ease.[6] Even warm bath water is enervating for these patients, many of whom felt very weak after taking a warm bath. Those living or vacationing in colder climates were more comfortable and more active than those who lived in warmer climates. Keeping your home on the cool side is recommended by these Belgian researchers.

Muscular Dystrophy

Whereas cool treatment helps Myasthenia Gravis, warmth is indicated for Muscular Dystrophy, even though both disturbances are a progressive degeneration of the body muscles. Again, nutrition can come to the rescue.

Animals, regardless of the type, if kept on a Vitamin E-deficient diet long enough, can develop muscular dystrophy. If the Vitamin E deficiency is caught early and corrected, the disturbance can be stopped in its tracks. But if the Vitamin E deficiency continues indefinitely, the disease may become irreversible. There is a test to pinpoint this deficiency. If creatine is found in the urine on laboratory testing, the disease is developing. However, if massive doses of Vitamin E plus concentrated wheat germ oil are given, plus protein, Vitamin A and Vitamin B-6 as well as all other B vitamins, degeneration may be controlled, and improvement, even recovery in some cases may occur.

Other medical findings for Muscular Dystrophy are encouraging. Professor Yoshito Takaoka, of Nagasaki University Medical School, Japan, found that a preparation of pancreatic enzyme could both improve and, in some cases, nearly reverse Muscular Dystrophy.

William H. Niedner, D.O. recommends massage to encourage circulation to weakened muscles. One three-year-old child, with no arm, leg or muscle strength, and unable to keep his food down, was eventually able to digest food as well as ride a tricycle, following regular massage.

A physician, Otakar Machek, M.D., after testing muscle strength with a myometer, and testing urine for creatine, found that minerals may not be properly assimilated by the body. He determined deficiencies of sodium, calcium, potassium, magnesium, phosphorus and chlorides in patients. When given in chelated form, these minerals were well assimilated,[7] and favorable results were obtained.

Anyone with symptoms of the neuromuscular group would be wise to not delay in checking diet. The earlier you begin, the better the chances for prevention or even reversal of these conditions. I have shared the nutritional tools with you. Now the rest is up to you.

Above all, maintain a cheerful outlook upon life and take your reverses as philosophically as possible. There is evidence that these neuromuscular diseases all appeared following severe, extended stress.

The late Dr. Henry A. Schroeder, who did so much work with trace elements, died of Muscular Dystrophy which he acquired early in his career. It was his strong belief that it is an hereditary disease.

REFERENCES
(See *Bibliography* for fuller details.)

1. Ebba Waerland, *Rebuilding Health*.
2. *International Journal of Environmental Studies*, Vol. 6, Part 1: 19–27; Part 2: 121–129, 1974.
3. *Clinica Chimica Acta*, May 15, 1975.
4. Adelle Davis, *Let's Get Well*.
5. Society for Experimental Biology and Medicine *Journal*, June, 1954.
6. *Lancet*, July 13, 1974
7. Sclerex tablets, available from Millar Pharmacal Co., Box 299, West Chicago, Ill. 60185, can be ordered through your doctor.

24: TEETH AND GUMS

Nearly everyone is beginning to accept the effect of nutrition on teeth and gums. Not only is it well known that sugar is a major cause of cavities, but also that sticky carbohydrates which cling to the teeth are suspect. Even so-called "healthful" sugars, such as dried fruits, are a problem, since foods like raisins, figs etc., eaten straight, stick to the teeth and are extremely high in sugar. Blackstrap molasses, a nutritionally superior food, when taken straight from the spoon, can cling to the teeth and erode them. Sharp, acidic juices, such as lemon and other citrus, have also been found to erode the enamel. The solution to this problem is easy: simply rinse the mouth or cleanse the teeth after each meal and immediately after taking the blackstrap, or citrus juices, so that they will not remain on the teeth and damage them. Fruits are less damaging than juices.

Few people may be aware of the deleterious effect of soft drinks. The late Dr. Clive McCay, of Cornell University, found in animal studies that, after constant exposure, the phosphoric acid in cola drinks dissolved teeth.

Gums react to nutrition, too. What you eat can make them firm or weak. And Dr. Juan M. Navia, Dental Research Professor, University of Alabama, states: "Nutrients may also affect the flow and composition of saliva in contact with plaque and enamel, and they can contribute to the composition of the outer enamel . . . good nutrition is the best ally preventive medicine or dentistry has. To lay aside such knowledge would be folly . . . ."

For gums which are already spongy, bleeding, or afflicted with any type of peridental disease, Vitamin C (ascorbic acid), but particularly the whole Vitamin C family or complex, known as the bioflavonoids, can help here. (It takes time, but it works.) This is both a treatment as well as a preventive measure. Periodontal disease is a low, insidious build-up of infection which causes the gums to become inflamed and the bony structures supporting the teeth to recede so that they can no longer hold the teeth in place. As a result, the teeth begin to loosen and fall out. In addition to the strengthening, tightening effect of ascorbic acid and the bioflavonoids, there is something still newer.

A team of researchers at the University of California, San Francisco, has discovered an exciting new help for those who suffer from shrinking gums and dental bones. The use of Vitamin E was given internally to fourteen periodontal patients. After three weeks, the fluid flow between the gingiva and the teeth (the measurement of the amount of inflammation present) had been reduced. The patients were told not to swallow the Vitamin E capsules whole, but to chew the gelatine capsules and rinse and swallow the enclosed remaining liquid.

The control group, given placebos (dummy pills), did not have the success provided by the Vitamin E. An acquaintance of mine went still further. She punctured a Vitamin E capsule and rubbed the contents on her gums before rinsing and swallowing. On her return to the dentist, he was amazed at the improvement.

Another helpful application is a Cayce liquid formula known as *Ipsab*. When Edgar Cayce first mentioned this substance in many readings, there was no such product on the market. It was necessary for him to come up with a formula, which he did, and it is now sold by a limited number of outlets stocking the Cayce remedies.[1] The formula is innocuous: "prickly ash" bark, salt, calcium chloride, peppermint and a certain nontoxic type of iodine. The readings suggested *Ipsab* for strengthening the gums; bleeding and receding gums; infections and pyorrhea; even preventing some of the more arduous efforts in root canal work (but as a preventive, not a reversal). *Ipsab* was also recommended by Edgar Cayce for developing healthy teeth in babies.

The method of using *Ipsab* is merely to apply it to the gums with the finger for massage. Some people rub it on their gums with a toothbrush. *Ipsab* has many devoted followers. I would not be without it.

Now that you know how to take care of your gums, what do you do about teeth which are already loose and when there is no time to lose before they begin to fall out? A study at Cornell reports great steps forward with this serious problem. Drs. Lennart Krook, D.V.M., Ph.D. and Leo Lutwalk, M.D., Ph.D found that ten dental patients, five men and five women between the ages of twenty-nine and forty-five, were suffering from a somewhat severe calcium deficiency. They had been taking only 400 mg. of calcium daily. The doctors corrected this situation by giving the patients for the next six months 1,000 mg. of calcium carbonate, in supplement form, daily.

At the beginning of the study, all patients had gingivitis (gum inflammation) and bleeding gums. After six months on the calcium therapy, the inflammation was improved in all cases, and completely gone in three. Loose teeth in eight patients were tighter in all but one case. As proof of the effect of this calcium therapy, *X-rays showed that healthy new bone had been deposited in the jaws of the patients given the calcium supplements.*[7] This is welcome news to dental patients who suffer from these conditions. Not only was bone resorption reversed, but the interior of the bone was found to be denser and stronger in a follow-up study of ninety patients.[3]

Why, do you suppose, that these results affected only the

majority of the ten patients? Why not ten out of ten? The answer may well be that taking calcium is not the only requirement. Many people may not assimilate it. Since acid in the body helps to dissolve the calcium and keep it in solution, where it can be in usable form by the body, *some* kind of acid must be taken with the calcium: Vitamin C, apple cider vinegar in water, or hydrochloric acid (available in tablet form at health stores).

And why calcium carbonate? There are many types of calcium. Calcium carbonate contains a constituent of bone, thus is compatible with bone and teeth. Milk, though high in calcium, causes trouble for some people who are allergic to it, as many are, especially cow's milk or milk products.

The Cornell researchers make a recommendation, based on their studies: most adults should take at least 1,100 mg. of calcium daily, plus magnesium and zinc, as protection against periodontal disease. But don't forget to assure your intake of sufficient acid (explained fully in my book, *Secrets of Health and Beauty*). Vitamin D either in supplemental form (tablets or perles, or cod liver oil) also helps calcium assimilation. Exposure to a little sun daily is another way of getting Vitamin D naturally. But don't overdo it.

There is a spectacular method of brushing teeth which is new. It was described in *Prevention* Magazine[4] by Dr. Stephen Feldman, Assistant Professor of Periodontics, and Coordinator of Preventive Dentistry Programs at the College of Medicine and Dentistry of New Jersey. Dr. Feldman refers to this toothbrushing method as the Bass technique. The patients to whom he recommended this method found that it stopped their gums from bleeding in about five days.

It is interesting to note Dr. Feldman's reaction to brushing in general. He not only quotes the statement of the American Society for Preventive Dentistry, "Even if you brush your teeth twice a day and see your dentist twice a year, this would not be enough to stop dental disease."

In fact, Dr. Feldman says you could brush fifty times a day and still get dental problems. This is because ordinary brushing does not usually remove plaque, which is an invisible, sticky, harmful bacterial deposit that forms on the teeth. But, if you brush your teeth once a day the *right way* (developed by Dr. Charles C. Bass, former Dean Emeritus of Tulane University Medical School), you can get rid of plaque. Here is the method:

1. Use the right type of brush, recommended by Dr. Bass. It should be a soft, rounded, "polished" or "satinized" nylon brush, safe for removing plaque.

2. To brush your upper teeth place the bristles at the gum line, at a 45° angle. Hold the bristles steady as you wiggle the brush vigorously back and forth. This helps to push the bristles through the crevices of the teeth.

3. Brush in a methodical manner. Do the outside of the teeth first, beginning at the gum line. After the wiggle of the brush, stroke the upper teeth downward, not sideways. Then repeat on the inside of the upper teeth, again beginning at the gum line. Do the front and back of the lower teeth in the same way, and after cleaning the teeth at the inside and outside gum level, stroke the teeth upward, or in the direction they grow. Rinse your mouth with warm water.

Do not worry if your gums bleed at first. They will soon harden up, Dr. Feldman states. And you will probably need to use dental floss as an auxiliary measure to remove particles of food between the teeth that the brush did not reach.

In addition to proper nutrition, adequate calcium, zinc and magnesium, there is one more piece of news about avoiding cavities. Dr. John N. Ott, together with two dentists, Drs. E. J. Amontree and J. W. Benfield, conducted a study in a Florida school which showed that use of newly developed fluorescent light, known as a full-spectrum fluorescent, and invented by Dr. Ott, President of the Environmental Health and Light Research Institute, Sarasota, Florida, reduced cavities in many children, as compared to the use of conventional fluorescent lighting. This new type of lighting is closer to natural sunlight, and is known as Vita-Lite. The Vita-Lite tubes fit into regulation fluorescent fixtures, and have been tested with animals as well as humans.

To date, good effects have been noted on eyes, skin and glandular response, with use of these lights, but this is the first time the effect of the lighting on teeth has been studied.

So you need not despair if your teeth are not behaving. As someone has wisely said, "Take care of your teeth, and they will take care of you."

REFERENCES

(See *Bibliography* for fuller details.)

1. Write for prices to The Heritage Store, Box 444, Virginia Beach, Va. 23458.
2. *Cornell Veterinarian*, January and July, 1972.
3. *Israel Journal of Medical Sciences*, 7:504–505, 1971.
4. *Prevention*, April, 1975.

BIBLIOGRAPHY

Abrahamson, E.M. and Pezet, A.W., *Body, Mind and Sugar*. New York, Henry Holt & Co., 1951.

Adams, Ruth and Murray, Frank, *Minerals, Kill or Cure?* New York, Larchmont Books, 1974.

Airola, Paavo O., N.D., *There is a Cure for Arthritis*. West Nyack, N. Y., Parker Publishing Co., 1968; Englewood Cliffs, N. J., Prentice-Hall, pb. ed.

———— *How to Get Well*. Phoenix, Ariz., Health Plus Publishers, 1974.

Berland, Theodore, M.D. and Snider, Gordon L., M.D., *Living With Your Bronchitis and Emphysema*. New York, St. Martin's Press, 1972.

Bicknell, Franklin, M.D. and Prescott, Frederick, M.Sc., *The Vitamins In Medicine*. Milwaukee, Lee Foundation for Nutritional Research.

Blume, Kathleen A., *Air Pollution in the Schools and Its Effect on Our Children*. Available from The Human Ecology Research Foundation, 120 N. Michigan Ave., Chicago, 211, 60611.

Brams, William A., M.D., *How to Live With Your Blood Pressure*. New York, Arco Publishing Co., 1974.

Campbell, Giraud W., D.O. with Stone, Robert, *A Doctor's Proven Cure for Arthritis*. West Nyack, N. Y., Parker Publishing Co., 1972.

Chapman, J. B., M.D., edited by Cogswell, J. W., M.D., *Dr. Schuessler's Biochemistry*. London, New Era Laboratories Ltd. (Available from Standard Homeopathic Pharmacy, P.O. Box 61067, Los Angeles, Cal. 90061.)

283

Cheraskin, E., M.D., D.M.D. and Ringsdorf, W.M. Jr., D.M.D., M.S., *Predictive Medicine.* Mountain View, Calif., Pacific Press Publishing Association, 1973.
——*New Hope for Incurable Diseases.* Hicksville, N. Y., Exposition Press, 1971.
——; Clark, J.W., D.D.S., *Diet and Disease.* Emmaus, Pa., Rodale Press, 1968.
——, with Arline Brecher, *Psychodietetics.* New York, Stein and Day, 1974.
Clark, Linda, *Are You Radioactive? How To Protect Yourself.* Old Greenwich, The Devin-Adair Co., 1973; New York, Pyramid Books, pb. ed.
——*Be Slim and Healthy.* New Canaan, Conn., Keats Publishing Co., 1972.
——*Color Therapy.* Old Greenwich, The Devin-Adair Co., 1975.
——*Get Well Naturally.* Old Greenwich, The Devin-Adair Co., 1967; New York, Arco Publishing Co., pb. ed., 1968.
——*Help Yourself to Health.* New York, Pyramid Books, 1972.
——*Know Your Nutrition.* New Canaan, Conn., Keats Publishing Co., 1973.
——*Secrets of Health and Beauty.* Old Greenwich, The Devin-Adair Co., 1969; New York, Pyramid Books, pb. ed., 1971.
——*Stay Young Longer.* New York, Pyramid Books, paperback, 1968.
Coca, Arthur F., M.D., *The Pulse Test.* New York, Arco Publishing Co.
Culpeper's Complete Herbal. English publication, distributed by Sterling Publishing Co., 419 Park Ave. So., New York, N. Y. 10016.

Davis, Adelle, *Let's Eat Right to Keep Fit.* New York, Harcourt Brace, 1954; New York, New American Library, Signet paperback.
——*Let's Get Well.* New York, New American Library, Signet paperback.
Di Cyan, Erwin, Ph.D., *Vitamins in Your Life and the Micronutrients.* New York, Simon & Schuster, 1972.

Eichenlaub, John E., M.D., *A Minnesota Doctor's Home Remedies for Common and Uncommon Ailments.* Englewood Cliffs, N. J., Prentice-Hall, 1960.
Ellis, John M., M.D., *The Doctor Who Looked at Hands.* New York, Arco Publishing Co., 19xx.
——"Review of Vitamin B-6," *Natural Food and Farming* magazine, June, 1970.
——, with Presley, James, *Vitamin B-6: The Doctor's Report,* New York, Harper & Row, 1973.
Elwood, Catharyn, *Feel Like A Million.* New York, Simon & Schuster, Pocket Books paperback, 1965.

Feingold, Ben F., M.D., *Introduction to Clinical Allergy.* Springfield, Ill., Charles C. Thomas, Publisher, 1973.

Fletcher, Horace, M.A., *Fletcherism, What It Is.* London, Ewart, Seymour & Co Ltd. Milwaukee, Lee Fndtn. for Nutritional Research, Am. ed.
Foley, Daniel J. and Miller, John J., Ph.D., monograph, "Alcoholism: A Threefold Disease." Available from Millar Pharmacal Company, Inc., P.O. Box 158, West Chicago, Ill. 60185.
Fredericks, Carlton, Ph.D. and Goodman, Herman, M.D., *Low Blood Sugar and You.* New York, Constellation International, 1969.
Friedman, Meyer, M.D. and Rosenman, Ray H., M.D., *Type A Behavior and Your Heart.* New York, Alfred A. Knopf, 1974.

Garten, M. O., M.D., *The Health Secrets of a Naturopathic Doctor.* West Nyack, N. Y., Parker Publishing Co., 1967.

Hackett, Clara A. with Galton, Lawrence, *Relax and See: A Daily Guide to Better Vision.* New York, Harpers, 1955; London, Faber & Faber, 1957.
Houston, F. M., D.C., *The Healing Benefits of Acupressure.* New Canaan, Conn., Keats Publishing Co., 1974.
Hurdle, J. Frank, M.D., *Doctor Hurdle's Program to Retain Youthfulness.* West Nyack, N. Y., Parker Publishing Co., 1972.

James, Claudia V., *That Old Green Magic.* Edmonton, Alberta, Canada, Amrita Books, 1952.
Jarvis, D. C., *Folk Medicine.* New York, Henry Holt & Co., 1958; New York, Fawcett-Crest, pb. ed.
———*Arthritis and Folk Medicine,* New York, Rinehart & Winston, 1960.
Jensen, Bernard, D.C., N.D., *The Science and Practice of Iridology.* Escondido, Calif., 1973.

Kadans, Joseph, N. D., Ph.D., *Modern Encyclopedia of Herbs.* West Nyack, New York, Parker Publishing Co., 1970.
——— *Encyclopedia of Medicinal Herbs.* New York, Arco Publishing Co., pb. ed., 1972.
Kaplan, Norman M., *Your Blood Pressure: The Most Deadly High.* New York, Medicom Press, 1974.
Kerner, Fred, *Dr. Hans Selye's Famous Concept of Stress and Your Heart.* New York, Hawthorne Books, 1961.
Kervran, Louis C., *Biological Transmutations.* Binghamton, N. Y., Swan House Publishing Co., 1972.
Korth, Leslie O., D.O., M.R.O., *Some Unusual Healing Methods.* Rustington, Sussex, England, Health Science Press, 1960.
Kroeger, Hanna, *Old-Time Remedies for Modern Ailments.* (Self-published, 7075 Valmont Drive, Boulder, Colorado.)

Lucas, Richard, *Common and Uncommon Uses of Herbs for Healthful Living.* New York, Arco Publishing Co., paperback.

———— *The Magic of Herbs in Daily Living.* West Nyack, N. Y., Parker Publishing Co., 1972.

Mességué, Maurice, *Of Men and Plants: The Autobiography of the World's Most Famous Plant Healer.* New York, The Macmillan Co., 1972.
———— *Way to Natural Health and Beauty.* New York, The Macmillan Co., 1974.

Nichols, Joe D., M.D., with Presley, James, *"Please Doctor, Do Something!"* Old Greenwich, The Devin-Adair Company, 1975.
Nittler, Alan H., M.D., *A New Breed of Doctor.* New York, Pyramid Books, 1974.
Nuramoto, Naboru, *Healing Ourselves.* Binghamton, N. Y., Swan House Publishing Co., 1973; New York, Avon Books, pb. ed., 1973.

Oliver, J. H., *Proven Remedies.* London, Thorson's Publishers Ltd., 12th edition, 1971.
Ott, John N., *Health and Light.* Old Greenwich, The Devin-Adair Co., 1973; New York, Simon & Schuster, Pocket Books pb. ed., 1976.
———— *My Ivory Cellar.* Old Greenwich, The Devin-Adair Co., 1971.

Page, Melvin E., D.D.S., *Degeneration to Regeneration,* St. Petersburg, Fla., Page Foundation, sixth printing, 1957.
———— *Anthropometrics.* St. Petersburg, Fla., Page Foundation, 1964.
Perry, Charles, *New Beauty,* Oshawa, Ont., Canada, Carley's Foods Ltd., Publishers.
Perry, Inez Eudora and Carey, George Washington, *The Zodiac and the Salts of Salvation,* New York, Samuel Weiser, Inc., 1971.
Pinckney, Edward R., M.D. and Cathey, *The Cholesterol Controversy.* Los Angeles, Sherbourne Press, 1973.
Potter's New Cyclopaedia. Rustington, Sussex, England, Health Science Press, 1971.
Price, Joseph M., M.D., *Coronaries, Cholesterol, Chlorine.* New York, Pyramid Books, 1971.

Randolph, Theron G., M.D., *Human Ecology and Susceptibility to the Chemical Environment.* Springfield, Ill., Charles C. Thomas, Publisher, 1962.
Richards, Guyon, M.D., *The Chain of Life.* Rustington, Sussex, England, Health Science Press, 1954.
Rodale, J. I. and Staff, *The Encyclopedia of Common Diseases.* Emmaus, Pa., Rodale Press, 1962.
———— *The Complete Book of Vitamins.* Emmaus, Pa., Rodale Press, 1966.
Rosenvold, Lloyd, M.D., *Drop Your Blood Pressure.* New York, Pyramid Books, 1974.
Rowe, A. H. Sr. and A. H. Jr., M.D.s, *Food Allergy.* Springfield, Ill., Charles C. Thomas, Publisher, 1972.

Samuels, Mike, M.D. and Bennett, Hal, *The Well Body Book.* New York, Random House, 1973.

Schroeder, Henry A., M.D., *The Trace Elements and Man.* Old Greenwich, The Devin-Adair Co., 1973.

Shute, Wilfrid E., M.D. with Taub, Harald J., *Vitamin E for Ailing and Healthy Hearts.* New York, Pyramid Books, paperback, 1972.

Silvers, Lewis J., *Extraordinary Remedies and Prescriptions for Health and Longevity.* Englewood Cliffs, N.J., Prentice-Hall, 1964.

Simpkins, R. Brooks, *Science and Our Eyes.* Eastbourne, Sussex, England, a pamphlet, 1972.

———*Visible Ray Therapy of the Eyes.* Rustington, Sussex, England, Health Science Press, 1963.

Stearn, Jess, *Edgar Cayce, The Sleeping Prophet.* New York, Doubleday & Co., 1967.

———*Dr. Thompson's New Way for You to Cure Your Aching Back.* New York, Doubleday & Co., 1973.

Sternglass, Ernest J., *Low Level Radiation.* New York, Ballantine Books, 1972.

Stone, Irwin, *The Healing Factor: Vitamin C Against Disease.* New York, Grosset & Dunlap, 1972.

Taub, Harald J., *Keeping Healthy in a Polluted World.* New York, Harper & Row, 1974.

Thienell, G. M., *My Battle With Low Blood Sugar.* Hicksville, N. Y., Exposition Press, 1970.

Tobe, John H., *Cataract, Glaucoma and Other Eye Disorders.* St. Catharine's, Ont., Canada, The Provoker Press, 1971.

"Victory Over Alcohol," a 32-page booklet of articles showing how faith can solve the problem. Introduction by Dr. Norman Vincent Peale. Available from *Guideposts,* Pawling, N.Y., 10512.

Waerland, Ebba, *Rebuilding Health.* New York, Arco Publishing Co., paperback, 1968.

Warmbrand, Max, N.D., D.O., D.C., *Overcoming Arthritis and Other Rheumatic Diseases.* Old Greenwich, The Devin-Adair Co., 1976.

Williams, Roger J., Ph.D., *Alcoholism, The Nutritional Approach.* Austin, University of Texas Press, 1951.

———A paper, "Broader Approach to the Prevention of Alcoholism", presented at the 12th International Institute on the Prevention and treatment of Alcoholism, Prague, Czechoslovakia, June 15, 1966.

———"Alcoholism, Malnutrition of the Brain," *Let's Live,* February, 1973.

Winter, Ruth, *Vitamin E, The Miracle Worker,* New York, Arco Publishing Co., paperback, 1972.

Yudkin, John, M.D., *Sweet and Dangerous.* New York, Peter H. Wyden Co., 1972.

INDEX